HEALING FOODS

55 Nutritious Foods
That Create Health, Balance Energy,
and Prevent Disease

Michio Kushi

Edited by Alex Jack
Illustrations by Bettina Zumdick

One Peaceful World Press
Becket, Massachusetts

Note to the Reader: Those with health problems are advised to seek the guidance of a qualified medical or nutritional professional before implementing any of the recommendations in this book. It is essential that any reader who has any reason to suspect serious illness seek appropriate advice. Neither this nor any other book should be used as a substitute for qualified care or treatment.

Healing Foods
Text © 1998 by Michio Kushi and Alex Jack
Illustrations © 1998 by Bettina Zumdick

For further information on mail-order sales, wholesale or retail discounts, distribution, translations, and foreign rights, please contact the publisher:

One Peaceful World Press
P.O. Box 10
Leland Road
Becket, MA 01223
U.S.A.

Telephone (413) 623-2322
Fax (413) 623-6042

First Edition: June 1998
10 9 8 7 6 5 4 3 2 1

ISBN 1–882984–31-5
Printed in U.S.A.

CONTENTS

KEY TO THE FOODS

The introductory paragraph describes the food's origin, use, and principal qualities.

Varieties & Use notes different varieties and forms of the food and how it is commonly used. Most foods are available in natural foods stores or from macrobiotic mail order companies. As much as possible, foods should be organic in quality.

Health benefits lists the major nutritional and energetic effects, especially on key organs, functions, and systems, including consciousness, as well as the use of the food in medicinal teas, compresses, plasters, or other external applications. Please see *Basic Home Remedies* by Michio Kushi (One Peaceful World Press, 1994) for further information.

Recipe includes a basic preparation for the food. Please see *Aveline Kushi's Complete Guide to Macrobiotic Cooking* by Aveline Kushi and Alex Jack (Warner Books, 1985) or other macrobiotic cookbook for further recipes and menus.

Cost presents the typical cost per pound or other unit of the food at the natural foods store. The price reflects the organic price, whenever available. Peak season of harvest or availability is also noted when appropriate.

Nutritional data lists the major nutrients of the raw (uncooked) food. Nutritional data is from the most recent U.S. Department of Agriculture *Standard Reference* (1997) or the *Standard Tables of Food Composition in Japan* (1998).

FOREWORD

Over the last generation, the macrobiotic and organic, natural foods movements have helped inspire a diet and health revolution in modern society. Today people are eating more whole grains, beans, fresh vegetables, sea vegetables, and other healthful foods than ever before. Rates of high blood pressure, heart disease, and even some forms of cancer have started to decline as a result, and a more comprehensive, holistic approach to mental and psychological health, family health, and the future of society is beginning to emerge.

Healing Foods profiles over fifty key foods that are beneficial to personal and planetary health as well as helping to prevent and relieve common ailments and diseases. They form the foundation of the modern macrobiotic way of eating and are increasingly available in supermarkets and restaurants, as well as natural foods stores and from mail-order companies.

Besides the foods described here, there are many other foods that are part of a balanced diet and which have healing properties. Please see the Appendix for an outline of the broad scope and variety of the Standard Macrobiotic Diet. In principle, all foods have medicinal effects based on their energetic effects and may be used under appropriate circumstances. The goal of macrobiotics is freedom, not restriction. The aim is to choose wisely, prepare food with a calm, peaceful mind, and be grateful for the great miracle of life.

In preparing this book, nutritional data have been taken primarily from the new U.S. government food tables. Please keep in mind that these tables are based on conventionally grown samples and that organic foods may be higher in some nutrients. However, since the last tables published in 1975, there has been a serious decline in mineral and vitamin content in many foods. This reflects a widespread loss in the quality of

5

soil, water, and air, as well as other environmental threats such as global warming and thinning of the ozone layer.

Meanwhile, genetically-altered foods, irradiated foods, and other artificial products have entered the marketplace. The absence of clear labeling means that most people are unaware when they are purchasing or eating these items. Proper labeling and freedom of choice in diet and food selection is a cornerstone of a healthy, free society. The U.S. government is currently introducing national organic standards for the first time, and this provides an opportunity to remedy this situation.

In preparing this volume, I am grateful to Alex Jack, director of One Peaceful World, for editing and preparing this book; to my wife, Aveline, and to Gale Jack, Alex's wife, for the recipes; Junji Oba, director of One Peaceful World Japan for supplying nutritional data of speciality foods from Japan; Virginia Chu and Laura Wepman for research and editorial assistance; Bettina Zumdick for the wonderful illustrations; and our many colleagues and students at the Kushi Institute, One Peaceful World, and around the globe who are working tirelessly to create a healthier, more peaceful planet.

Michio Kushi
Brookline, Massachusetts
May 17, 1998

AGAR AGAR

Agar agar is a traditional sea vegetable product available in the form of translucent bars, powder, flakes, or strands and is used in cooking as a gelatin or setting agent.

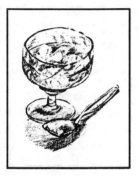

Varieties & Use: Agar is derived from red algae found in Japanese waters, other Pacific regions, and the Atlantic. Agar is dissolved in hot liquid, poured over cooked fruit, and allowed to cool into a delicious gelatin dish called *kanten*, or put over beans or vegetables to form an *aspic*. It may also be prepared plain with a miso or shoyu sauce, grated ginger, or chopped scallions.

Health Benefits: Agar agar is an excellent source of iodine (160 mg per 100 grams compared to 0.07 mg for a typical serving of fish). Agar agar is particularly soothing for the intestines and is used to improve digestion and the bowels.

Recipe for Kanten: In a pot, bring 2 cups of spring water, 2 cups of apple juice, and a pinch of sea salt to a boil, gradually stirring in 1 bar or 4 Tbsp. of agar until it dissolves. Reduce heat, simmer for 15 min. Add slices of 3 apples the last 5 min., stirring occasionally. Pour into large dish or individual molds. Refrigerate until jelled, usually 45-60 minutes.

Cost: $4.00/1-oz. package; year-round

Composition of Agar Agar, 100 Grams, Edible Portion

Water	Calories	Protein	Fat	Carbo.	Fiber	Calcium	Phos.
8.7 gm.	306	6.2 gm.	0.3 gm.	80.9 gm.	7.7 gm.	625 mg.	52 mg.
Iron	Sodium	Potass.	Vit. A	Thiamin	Ribofla.	Niacin	Vit. C
21.4 mg.	102 mg.	1125 mg	0	0.01 mg.	0.22 mg.	0.2 mg.	0

AMASAKE

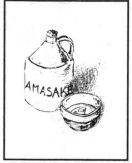

Amasake is a delicious rice-based sweetener made from sweet brown rice and *koji*, a bacterial starter, that are allowed to ferment into a thick liquid. As a beverage or sweetener, amasake has a rich, satisfying taste and creamy, thick texture.

Varieties & Use: Amasake may be made at home or be purchased ready-made in natural food stores. Store-bought amasake is available plain or flavored with almonds, apricot, mocha, or other ingredients. Amasake is used as a sweetener for puddings, pies, cakes, and other desserts. It is also served warm or chilled as a porridge or beverage. It may be enjoyed by itself or topped with strawberries, other fruit, or grated ginger.

Health Benefits: Amasake is a high quality natural sweetener and gives strong energy. It is traditionally used by nursing mothers, babies, and others needing strength and vitality. It is also used to help offset tight, contractive conditions.

Recipe for Amasake Pudding: Combine 1 qt. amasake with 6 Tbsp. of kuzu diluted in a little cold water in a pot. Stir slowly, bring to a boil, simmer 2-3 min., and pour into serving dishes. Garnish with lemon and parsley, let set, and serve.

Cost: $2.00-3.00/16-oz. bottle; year-round

Composition of Amasake, 100 Grams, Edible Portion

Water 74.0 gm.	Calories 104	Protein 2.4 gm.	Fat 0.1 gm.	Carbo. 22.7 gm.	Fiber 0.6 gm.	Calcium 2 mg.	Phos. 25 mg.
Iron 0.4 mg.	Sodium 2.0 mg	Potass. 10 mg.	Vit. A 0	Thiamin 0.01 mg.	Ribofla. 0.03 mg.	Niacin 0.2 mg.	Vit. C 0

ARAME

A dark sea vegetable native to Asian, South American, and European coastal waters, ara-me is enjoyed for its sweet, delicate taste and mild texture.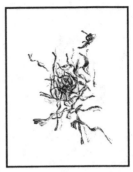

Varieties & Use: After being harvested, arame is dried and shredded, forming a mass of wiry black threads. When cooked, arame turns dark brown. Arame is frequently sautéed with carrots, onions, burdock, or other vegetables; tofu or tempeh; or dried daikon and served as a side dish. It is also delightful in soups and salads.

Health Benefits: As an excellent source of plant-quality iron and calcium, arame is good for the teeth and bones. It is also beneficial for the circulatory system and is used as an external home remedy for women's reproductive problems (as a substitute for daikon leaves in a *hip bath*).

Recipe for Arame with Onions: Wash and drain 1 oz. of arame. Sauté 2 sliced onions for 2-3 minutes. Add arame and enough water to cover the onions. Bring to a boil, lower heat, add 1 Tbsp. shoyu. Cover, simmer 40-50 minutes, add more shoyu to taste, simmer another 15-20 minutes. Mix and stir until liquid is evaporated and serve.

Cost: $3.50-4.00/1.76-2-oz. package; year-round

Composition of Arame, 100 Grams, Edible Portion

Water 9.7 gm.	Calories --	Protein 8.0 gm.	Fat 0.1 gm.	Carbo. 54.1 gm.	Fiber 10.4 gm.	Calcium 830 mg	Phos. 220 mg.
Iron 5.1 mg.	Sodium 2900 mg	Potass. 3700 mg	Vit. A 190 I.U.	Thiamin 0.06 mg.	Ribofla. 0.37 mg.	Niacin 2.0 mg.	Vit. C 0

AZUKI BEANS

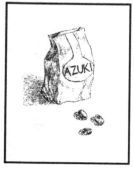

Azuki beans (also spelled *aduki*) are small, oval-shaped red or brown beans traditionally eaten in the Far East and now cultivated in the U.S. and elsewhere.

Varieties & Use: Azuki beans are enjoyed as a small side dish, cooked with brown rice to make *red rice*, used in soup, or prepared with agar agar as an aspic. Azukis are also a principal ingredient of a dish prepared with butternut or buttercup squash and kombu. They are also used to coat *ohagis* (sweet rice balls).

Health Benefits: Azuki beans contain less fat and oil than other beans. They are beneficial to the kidney, bladder, and reproductive functions and are used in medicinal dishes and drinks. Azukis also contribute to smooth bowel movements.

Recipe for Azuki Beans and Squash: Wash 1 cup azukis, cover with water, soak 6-8 hrs. Put a 6-8 inch strip of kombu in a pot and cover with 1 cup cubed winter squash. Add the azukis, cover with water to the level of the squash. Bring to a slow boil, cover, cook 1 hour, adding cold water if necessary to keep water level constant and soften beans. When 70-80% done, add 1/4 tsp sea salt, cook another 15-30 min. until liquid evaporates.

Cost: $2.00/lb. domestic, $5.50/lb.; Hokkaido; year-round

Composition of Japanese Azukis, 100 Grams, Edible Portion

Water 15.5 gm.	Calories 339	Protein 20.3 gm.	Fat 2.2 gm.	Carbo. 54.4 gm.	Fiber 4.3 gm.	Calcium 75 mg.	Phos. 350 mg.
Iron 5.4 mg.	Sodium 1.0 mg.	Potass. 1500 mg	Vit. A 0	Thiamin 0.45 mg	Ribofla. 0.16 mg.	Niacin 2.2 mg.	Vit. C 0

BANCHA TWIG TEA

Bancha twig tea ("late growing tea," also known as *kukicha*) is harvested from the twigs of the tea bush and is the main daily beverage in many Far Eastern, macrobiotic, and natural foods households.

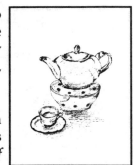

Varieties & Use: Various grades of bancha twig tea are available in the natural foods store. These are different from *bancha leaf tea* or *green tea* which is made from the leaves of the tea bush or dyed *black tea*.

Health Benefits: Bancha twig tea has a soothing, beneficial effect on digestion, blood quality, and the mind. It is safe for children and infants to drink. Because the caffeine in the tea bush recedes from the twigs, it has virtually no caffeine or tannin. Nor does it have an aromatic, stimulating effect like most herbal teas. Loaded with calcium, iron, and vitamins A and C, bancha twig tea has many medicinal uses, ranging from *ume-sho-bancha tea* for alkalizing the blood and relieving fatigue to an external compress for eye conditions.

Basic Bancha Twig Tea: Place 1 1/2-2 Tbsp. twigs in 1 1/2 qts. spring water and bring to a boil. Reduce heat, simmer for 2-3 min. for light tea or 10 min. for a strong tea. Strain and serve.

Cost: Loose Twigs $6.00/8 oz.; 20 Tea Bags $3.75; year-round

Composition of Twig Tea (brewed), 100 Grams, Edible Portion

Water	Calories	Protein	Fat	Carbo.	Fiber	Calcium	Phos.
4.4 gm.	--	19.7 gm.	4.4 gm.	33.5 gm.	19.5 gm.	740 mg.	210 mg.
Iron	Sodium	Potass.	Vit. A	Thiamin	Ribofla.	Niacin	Vit. C
38.0 mg.	4 mg.	1900 mg	7800 IU.	0.25 mg.	1.4 mg.	5.4 mg.	150 mg.

BARLEY

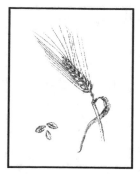

Barley, the ancient grain and traditional staple of Southern Europe, North Africa, and the Middle East, is grown around the world and is a major cereal crop.

Varieties & Use: *Whole* or *hulled barley* is the most nutritious. *Pearled barley* is a partially processed form, while *pearl barley* is another cereal grain altogether (see *Hato Mugi*). Roasted barley is used to make a soothing tea, *mugi cha*. Barley is used to make *mugi miso*. Barley *malt* is used as a natural sweetener in desserts and baked goods. Barley is enjoyed in thick, delicious soups and stews. It is also cooked with other grains, beans, or vegetables (e.g., as stuffing for cabbage or squashes).

Health Benefits: Barley produces a light, cooling effect. It is especially beneficial for the liver and gallbladder. Soft barley or barley gruel was the principal home remedy in the early Western medical tradition. Barley may be mixed with tofu to form a *barley/tofu plaster* used to reduce inflammation.

Recipe for Soft Barley: Combine 1 cup barley, 4-5 cups of spring water, and pinch of sea salt in a pot and boil for 1 1/4-1 1/2 hours. Garnish with scallions, parsley, nori, or gomashio.

Cost: Hulled $.50-.1.00/lb.; year-round

Composition of Barley, 100 Grams, EdiblePortion

Water	Calories	Protein	Fat	Carbo.	Fiber	Calcium	Phos.
9.4 gm.	354	12.5 gm.	2.3 gm.	73.5 gm.	17.3 gm.	33 mg.	264 mg.
Iron	Sodium	Potass.	Vit. A	Thiamin	Ribofla.	Niacin	Vit. E
3.6 mg.	12.0 mg.	452 mg.	22 I.U.	0.6 mg.	0.3 mg.	4.6 mg.	0.6 mg.

BOK CHOY

Bok choy is a long cabbage-like vegetable with a wide white stalk and tender, dark green leaves. A traditional ingredient in Chinese cooking, bok choy (also known as *pak choy, pak choi,* and *white mustard cabbage*) is now grown around the world and prized for its mild taste and light, crisp texture.

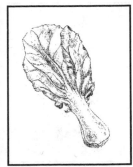

Varieties & Use: Bok choy is available in natural foods stores, Oriental markets, and many supermarkets. Bok choy blends well with other vegetables as well as fried tofu, tempeh, fish, seafood, or other strong-tasting foods. It may be sautéed, steamed, or boiled and be served with a kuzu sauce.

Health Benefits: Like other leafy green vegetables, bok choy is especially beneficial for the liver and gallbladder. It is high in calcium, iron, and other minerals.

Recipe for Sautéed Bok Choy: Sauté thinly sliced bok choy in a little sesame oil for 3-5 minutes. Add a few drops of shoyu, cover for 1-2 minutes, and serve.

Cost: $1.00-2.00/pound; peak, spring/summer

Composition of Bok Choy, 100 Grams, Edible Portion

Water	Calories	Protein	Fat	Carbo.	Fiber	Calcium	Phos.
95.3 gm.	13	1.5 gm.	0.2 gm.	2.2 gm.	1.0 gm.	105 mg.	37 mg.
Iron	Sodium	Potass.	Vit. A	Thiamin	Ribofla.	Niacin	Vit. C
0.8 mg.	65 mg.	252 mg.	3000 IU.	0.04 mg.	0.07 mg.	0.5 mg.	45 mg.

BROCCOLI

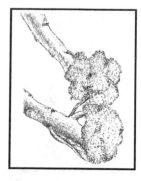

Broccoli's mild taste, attractive shape, bright green color, and firm, crisp texture make it a popular vegetable worldwide.

Varieties & Use: Broccoli is Italian for "cabbage sprout." Available year round, it peaks in the fall and spring and sometimes has a purple hue. Broccoli is prepared in a variety of ways, including light boiling (to retain its bright color), steaming, sautéing, tempura-style, or in shishkebob. It may also be lightly pickled or marinated for quick salads. It is especially delicious with fried rice, fried noodles, or mixed vegetables. A creamy tofu dressing, an umeboshi sauce, roasted sesame seeds, or other dressing is frequently served.

Health Benefits: Broccoli is beneficial to all major functions and organs, particularly the lungs and large intestine. High in fiber, beta carotene, calcium, and vitamin C, broccoli lowers the risk of cancer and heart disease.

Recipe for Broccoli with Tofu Dressing: Simmer 1 head of broccoli, cut into flowerets and stems, in a little water for 2-3 min. Squeeze out water from 1 lb. tofu, add 1-2 pitted umeboshi plums, and purée until smooth and creamy. Serve together.

Cost: $1.00-2.00/lb.; peak summer

Composition of Broccoli, 100 Grams, Edible Portion

Water	Calories	Protein	Fat	Carbo.	Fiber	Calcium	Phos.
90.7 gm.	28	3.0 gm.	0.4 gm.	5.2 gm.	3.0 gm.	48 mg.	66 mg.
Iron	Sodium	Potass.	Vit. A	Thiamin	Ribofla.	Niacin	Vit. C
0.9 mg.	27 mg.	325 mg.	1542 IU.	0.07 mg	0.12 mg.	0.6 mg.	93 mg.

BROWN RICE

From South China, Southeast Asia, and Africa, rice has spread around the world.

Varieties and Use: *Short-grain rice* contains small kernels and is grown in temperate latitudes; *long-grain*, contains larger kernels and is produced in warmer regions; and *medium-grain* is in between. *Sweet rice* is a glutinous variety and *basmati* a long-grain rice native to the tropics. The bran, germ, 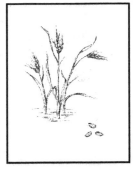 and other nutritious layers have been removed from *white rice*. Brown rice has a nutty flavor and chewy texture. It is pressure-cooked or boiled as the main dish in the meal; cooked with a small amount of beans, seeds, or nuts; steamed; fried; or made into croquettes, rice balls, or sushi.

Health Benefits: Brown rice contains a nearly perfect balance of energy and nutrients. Brown rice gives strong energy, a calm, clear mind, and sound judgment. It also has traditionally been eaten to develop unity and spiritual awareness.

Recipe for Pressure-Cooked Brown Rice: Wash 2 cups of rice, place in presssure cooker, add 3 cups spring water, and bring to pressure. Add pinch or two of sea salt when water starts to boil, tighten cover, bring to pressure, and cook for 50 minutes.

Cost: $1.25/1 lb.; $7.50/5 lbs.; $30.00/25 lb.; year-round

Composition of Brown Rice 100 Grams, Edible Portion

Water	Calories	Protein	Fat	Carbo.	Fiber	Calcium	Phos.
12.4 gm.	362	7.5 gm.	2.7 gm.	76.2 gm.	3.4 gm.	33 mg.	264 mg.
Iron	Sodium	Potass.	Vit. A	Thiamin	Ribofla.	Niacin	Vit. E
1.8 mg.	4.0 mg.	268 mg.	0	0.4 mg.	0.04 mg.	4.3 mg.	0.7 mg.

BUCKWHEAT

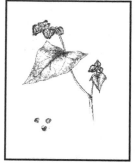

Buckwheat, the hardiest of the cereal plants, is a traditional staple in Russia, Eastern Europe, and parts of central and northern Asia. From the Far East, the popularity of buckwheat noodles has spread worldwide.

Varieties & Use: Buckwheat kernels are called *groats* and they are usually eaten in whole form or in coarse or fine granules and prepared as *kasha*. Buckwheat noodles, containing from 40 to 100% buckwheat, are known as *soba*. The deep, rich taste of buckwheat flour also makes tasty dumplings, muffins, pancakes, and waffles.

Health Benefits: Buckwheat gives strong, warming energy and is excellent as a preparation for hard, physical labor. It is used medicinally for weak, expansive disorders, but contraindicated for strong, contractive ones. A *buckwheat plaster* is good for drawing excess liquid from the body.

Recipe for Kasha: Wash 1 cup buckwheat, dry-roast for several minutes, put in pot, add 2 cups boiling water, and a pinch or two of sea salt. Bring to a boil, lower the heat, simmer for 20-30 minutes or until water is absorbed. Garnish with parsley.

Cost: $.65-.75/lb.; year-round

Composition of Buckwheat, 100 Grams, Edible Portion

Water 9.8 gm.	Calories 343	Protein 13.3 gm.	Fat 3.4 gm.	Carbo. 71.5 gm.	Fiber 10.0 gm.	Calcium 18 mg.	Phos. 347 mg.
Iron 2.2 mg.	Sodium 1.0 mg.	Potass. 560 mg.	Vit. A 0	Thiamin 0.1 mg	Ribofla. 0.4 mg.	Niacin 7.0 mg.	Vit. E 1.0 mg.

BURDOCK

Burdock is a long, thin root vegetable, dark brown in color, and firm in texture.

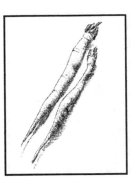

Varieties & Use: Wild burdock is frequently found in urban areas as well as the countryside. Domesticated varieties are available in the natural foods store. Burdock is sautéed kinpira-style with carrots, lotus root, or other root vegetables, It may also be boiled, steamed, or deep-fried. It blends well with grains, beans, and kombu but not hiziki or arame.

Health Benefits: Burdock gives strong energy and is excellent for weak, expansive conditions. It is good for the lungs and large intestines, helps alkalize the blood and bodily fluids, and strengths sexual functioning. In the Far East, *koi-koku*, a soup made with burdock, carp, miso, and bancha tea, is used to increase energy and restore vitality.

Recipe for Burdock Kinpira: Place 1 cup burdock, shaved or cut into matchsticks, in pan and sauté for 2-3 minutes in 1 tsp of dark sesame oil. Add 2 cups carrots, cut into matchsticks, and sauté for another 2-3 min. Add water to half cover the vegetables, season with shoyu, bring to a boil, reduce heat, cover, and simmer for 30 min. or until all the liquid has evaporated.

Cost: Fresh $2.00-5.00/lb.; Dried $6.00/4 oz.; year-round

Composition of Burdock, 100 Grams, Edible Portion

Water 80.1 gm.	Calories 72	Protein 1.5 gm.	Fat 0.2 gm.	Carbo. 17.4 gm.	Fiber 3.3 gm.	Calcium 47 mg.	Phos. 71 mg.
Iron 0.8 mg.	Sodium 5.0 mg.	Potass. 308 mg.	Vit. A 0	Thiamin 0.01 mg.	Ribofla. 0.03 mg.	Niacin 0.3 mg.	Vit. C 3 mg.

CABBAGE

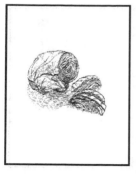

Cabbage has been eaten in Europe and Asia for thousands of years and is valued for its mild, crisp texture and natural sweet taste.

Varieties & Use: There are many forms and varieties, including round, conical, and flat, with compact or loose heads, smooth or curly leaves, and colors ranging from green to purple and red. Cabbage is enjoyed in soups, salads, and stir-fries. It may also be stuffed with couscous or rice, filled with tempeh, tofu, seitan, arame, or hijiki, or used for sauerkraut.

Health Benefits: Cabbage's sweet taste and balanced energy are good for the pancreas, spleen, and stomach. High in vitamins A and C, green cabbage is used in sweet vegetable drink and other medicinal preparations. As an external remedy, cabbage leaves or a *chlorophyll plaster* will reduce fever, neutralize inflammation, or relieve burns and bruises.

Recipe for Boiled Cabbage with Sesame and Umeboshi Sauce: Boil 4 cups thinly sliced cabbage in 2 cups of spring water for 2-3 minutes. Drain the cabbage and add 2 tsp. of kuzu diluted in a little cold water and 1-2 umeboshi plums for the sauce. Mix in sauce and add roasted sesame seeds on top.

Cost: $.75-1.00/lb.; peak autumn-winter

Composition of Cabbage, 100 Grams, Edible Portion

Water 92.2 gm.	Calories 25	Protein 1.4 gm.	Fat 0.3 gm.	Carbo. 5.4 gm.	Fiber 2.3 gm.	Calcium 47 mg.	Phos. 23 mg.
Iron 0.6 mg.	Sodium 18 mg.	Potass. 246 mg.	Vit. A 133 I.U.	Thiamin 0.05 mg	Ribofla. 0.04 mg.	Niacin 0.3 mg.	Vit. C 32.2 mg.

CARROT

Carrot's bright orange color, firm texture, and sweet taste are enjoyed around the world.

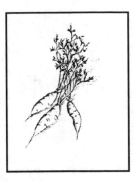

Varieties & Use: One of the most versatile vegetables, carrots are used in salads, soups (including carrot soup, miso soup, and mixed vegetable soups), stir-fries, and casseroles. They blend especially well with other root vegetables and sea vegetables. Carrot juice is very refreshing. Pickled carrots, carrot tempura, and carrot cake are also enjoyable. *Carrot tops* may be cooked and are a nutritious green.

Health Benefits: As a root vegetable, carrot's high beta-carotene and mild downward energy are especially good for the lungs and large intestine, as well as liver, kidneys, and heart. Medicinally, it is used in *carrot-daikon drink, sweet vegetable drink,* and as a substitute for burdock in *koi-koku.*

Recipe for Carrot Soup: Place 3 cups of grated carrots and 1 cup of minced onions in a pot. Add 5-6 cups of spring water and a pinch of sea salt. Bring to a boil, reduce heat, cover, and simmer for 20-25 min. Add another pinch or two of sea salt, simmer for 10-15 min., garnish with scallions or nori, and serve.

Cost: $.75-1.25/lb.; peak autumn-winter

Composition of Carrot, 100 Grams, Edible Portion

Water	Calories	Protein	Fat	Carbo.	Fiber	Calcium	Phos.
87.7 gm.	43	1.0 gm.	0.2 gm.	10.1 gm.	3.0 gm.	27 mg.	44 mg.
Iron	Sodium	Potass.	Vit. A	Thiamin	Ribofla.	Niacin	Vit. C
0.5 mg.	35.0 mg.	323 mg.	28129 IU	0.10 mg.	0.06 mg.	0.9 mg.	9.3 mg.

CAULIFLOWER

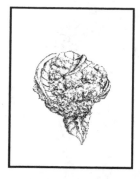

Cauliflower has a beautiful white color, flowery shape, crispy texture, sweet taste, and mild, calming energy.

Varieties & Use: White cauliflower is the most common, but purple and green are also available. As an appetizer (raw, marinated, or lightly boiled), cauliflower is tasty. It may also be pickled (whole or sliced) with shoyu and rice vinegar. Boiled cauliflower is enjoyed with a shoyu-lemon-ginger sauce or with an umeboshi vinegar sauce and roasted sesame seeds. Thickened with kuzu root, cauliflower makes a creamy, delicious soup. With millet, it makes millet mashed potatoes.

Health Benefits: Cauliflower is beneficial for the lungs and large intestine. High in vitamin C and beta-carotene, it is known to help prevent cancer and heart disease as part of a balanced diet.

Recipe for Boiled Cauliflower with a Lemon-Shoyu Sauce: Place a very small amount of spring water in a pot and bring to a boil. Add 2 cups of cauliflower flowerets and stems, cover, and boil until done, about 5 min. Serve with sauce made from water, shoyu, grated fresh ginger, and fresh lemon.

Cost: $1.00-1.50/lb..; peak summer-autumn

Composition of Cauliflower, 100 Grams, Edible Portion

Water 91.9 gm.	Calories 25	Protein 2.0 gm.	Fat 0.2 gm.	Carbo. 5.2 gm.	Fiber 2.5 gm.	Calcium 22 mg.	Phos. 44 mg.
Iron 0.4 mg.	Sodium 30 mg.	Potass. 303 mg.	Vit. A 19 I.U.	Thiamin 0.06 mg	Ribofla. 0.06 mg.	Niacin 0.5 mg.	Vit. C 46.4 mg.

CHICKPEAS

Chickpeas are small, hard, compact, and have a sweet taste and soothing energy.

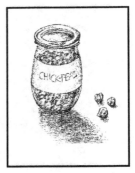

Varieties & Use: In Spanish, chickpeas are called *garbanzos* and are sometimes sold under this name. Cooked and ground into a paste and mixed with lemon, oil, and tahini, chickpeas make a tasty spread called *hummus*. Chickpeas make an appetizing side dish or may be cooked with brown rice or other grain. They go well with celery, carrots, and corn or mixed vegetables. They can be pan-fried into patties mixed and mashed with seitan.

Health Benefits: Like other high-fiber foods, chickpeas are excellent to help lower cholesterol. High in protein, minerals, and B vitamins, they are strengthening for the kidneys and bladder.

Recipe for Chickpeas with Vegetables: After soaking for several hours, pressure cook 1 cup chickpeas with a 3-inch piece of kombu for 45 minutes. Let pressure come down, add 1 small carrot, diced, 1 small onion, diced, 1/2 cup parsnips, sliced, and 1 cup cabbage, chopped, and pinch of sea salt. Cook 10 minutes more or until vegetables are tender. Add 1 Tbsp. barley miso at end and simmer gently for 4-5 minutes.

Cost: $1.50-2.00/lb.; year-round

Composition of Chickpeas, 100 Grams, Edible Portion

Water 11.5 gm.	Calories 364	Protein 19.3 gm.	Fat 6.0 gm.	Carbo. 60.7 gm.	Fiber 17.4 gm.	Calcium 105 mg.	Phos. 366 mg.
Iron 6.2 mg.	Sodium 24 mg.	Potass. 875 mg.	Vit. A 67 I.U.	Thiamin 0.48 mg.	Ribofla. 0.21 mg.	Niacin 1.5 mg.	Vit. C 4 mg.

COLLARD GREENS

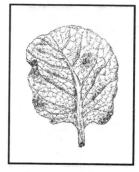

Collard greens, a traditional Native American, African-American, and Southern delicacy, have moved into the mainstream. Tender, sweet, and mild, the freshest varieties melt in the mouth.

Varieties & Use: Collards grow readily in gardens in the North as well as South. Collards may be lightly boiled or steamed for a few minutes and go well with a shoyu-rice vinegar sauce. The stalks may be thinly sliced and cooked at the same time.

Health Benefits: High in vitamins A and C, as well as calcium and other minerals, collards are especially strengthening for the liver, gallbladder, heart, and small intestine. Collards may be used to make *leafy greens juice* to treat liver disorders and dissolve heavy, stagnated protein, animal fat, or cholesterol. Their large green leaves are used in a *chlorophyll plaster* to reduce fever, sooth inflammation, or relieve burns.

Recipe for Steamed Collards with Shoyu-Vinegar Sauce: Steam 3 cups of thinly sliced collards in a small amount of water for several minutes, keeping the greens bright green. Mix shoyu, brown rice vinegar, and spring water to make a sauce.

Cost: $1.50-2.00/lb.; peak January-April

Composition of Collard Greens, 100 Grams, Edible Portion

Water 90.6 gm.	Calories 30	Protein 2.5 gm.	Fat 0.4 gm.	Carbo. 5.7 gm.	Fiber 3.6 gm.	Calcium 145 mg.	Phos. 10 mg.
Iron 0.2 mg.	Sodium 20 mg.	Potass. 169 mg.	Vit. A 3824 IU.	Thiamin 0.05 mg	Ribofla. 0.13 mg.	Niacin 0.7 mg.	Vit. C 35.3 mg.

CORN

Native to Central and South America, corn (or *maize*) is one of the most versatile cereal crops. Eaten on the cob, ground into whole corn dough, or made into grits, flour, or oil, corn is a staple for hundreds of millions of people around the world.

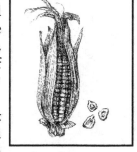

Varieties & Use: *Sweet corn* is the most common variety, while *dent, flour, flint*, and *popcorn* are also available. *Masa* is sold in some natural foods stores and can be made at home. *Open-pollinated* or *standard corn* is preferred to hybrid varieties. Avoid genetically-engineered corn, as well as cornmeal, corn starch, and refined corn oil (*unrefined oil* is suitable). Corn is enjoyed in soups, salads, cooked with rice or other grain, added to stir-fries, eaten in the form of polenta, tacos, tostadas, arepas, empanadas, cornbread, and other traditional dishes.

Health Benefits: Corn provides light, expansive energy and is especially strengthening for the heart and small intestine.

Recipe for Baked Corn on the Cob: Put 4-8 ears of fresh corn, in their husks, on a baking sheet and bake in a preheated 350-degree oven for 30 min. Remove husks and serve with condiment made from puréeing 1-2 umeboshi plums with water.

Cost: $.25-.50/ear; peak summer-autumn

Composition of Corn, 100 Grams, Edible Portion

Water	Calories	Protein	Fat	Carbo.	Fiber	Calcium	Phos.
76.0 gm.	86	3.2 gm.	1.2 gm.	19.0 gm.	2.7 gm.	2.0 mg.	89 mg.
Iron	Sodium	Potass.	Vit. A	Thiamin	Ribofla.	Niacin	Vit. C
0.5 mg.	15 mg.	270 mg.	281 I.U.	0.2 mg.	0.06 mg.	1.7 mg.	6.8 mg.

DAIKON

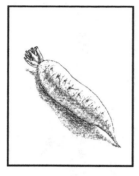

Daikon ("big root," also known as Oriental radish or white radish) is a major ingredient in Far Eastern cuisine and medicine and now popular in the West.

Varieties & Use: The large, juicy ones are sweet, while the small, thin ones have a strong, sharp taste. *Daikon leaves* make a delicious side dish. *Dried daikon* is also sweet. Daikon is enjoyed boiled, steamed, or pickled. It goes well with other root vegetables, beans, deep-fried or dried tofu, tempeh, shiitake mushrooms, and other ingredients. *Grated daikon* aids in digesting tempura, fish, or mochi.

Health Benefits: Daikon has strong dissolving energy and helps to digest fat and oil, as well as discharge animal products from the past. Medicinally, it is used in teas and plasters. Daikon leaves are used in a *hip bath* to alleviate women's reproductive organs and skin troubles.

Recipe for Boiled Daikon: Place 2 strips of sliced kombu in a pot. Layer 1 medium daikon, cut into 1/2-inch rounds, add water to half cover, and bring to a boil. Cover, reduce heat, simmer until translucent and soft, about 30-40 minutes. Season with miso diluted in a little water for 3-5 minutes more.

Cost: Fresh $1.00-1.50/lb.; Dried, $4.00-5.00/3.5 oz.; year-round

Composition of Fresh Daikon, 100 Grams, Edible Portion

Water	Calories	Protein	Fat	Carbo.	Fiber	Calcium	Phos.
94.6 gm.	18	0.6 gm.	0.1 gm.	4.1 gm.	1.6 gm.	27 mg.	23 mg.
Iron	Sodium	Potass.	Vit. A	Thiamin	Ribofla.	Niacin	Vit. C
0.4 mg.	21 mg.	227 mg.	0	0.02 mg	0.02 mg.	0.2 mg.	22 mg.

GINGER ROOT

Ginger, a light golden root, has a knobby form, pungent taste, and firm texture. It is a versatile garnish and medicinal food.

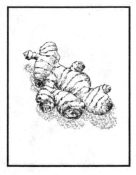

Varieties & Use: Fresh ginger is widely available, but *powdered ginger* may be substituted. Ginger is grated and added to grain and vegetable dishes, soups, salads, or sea vegetables and cooked for a few minutes just prior to serving. It is used as a garnish for sushi, tempura, fish, seafood, and other oily foods. Grated ginger is used to make a ginger compress.

Health Benefits: Ginger gives warmth to the body and adds richness to many dishes. Its strong, dispersing energy is used medicinally in teas, *ginger compress*, *body scrub*, and other internal and external applications to promote circulation, dissolve stagnation, and stimulate *Ki* energy flow. Mixed with sesame oil, it is used to relieve scalp, eye, ear, or arthritic ailments.

Recipe for Lemon-Ginger Pickles: Mince 10 lemon peels and put in pot with 1/2 cup spring water. Cook uncovered for 5 minutes. Sauté the cooked lemon peel, 1 cup of miso, and 1 tsp. of grated fresh ginger. Mix thoroughly and cook for 2-3 minutes. Cool, store in a jar for 1 week, and serve with rice or salad.

Cost: $2.00-3.00/lb.; year-round

Composition of Ginger Root, 100 Grams, Edible Portion

Water 81.7 gm.	Calories 69	Protein 1.7 gm.	Fat 0.7 gm.	Carbo. 15.1 gm.	Fiber 2.0 gm.	Calcium 18 mg.	Phos. 27 mg.
Iron 0.5 mg.	Sodium 13 mg.	Potass. 415 mg.	Vit. A 0	Thiamin 0.02 mg.	Ribofla. 0.03 mg.	Niacin 0.7 mg.	Vit. C 5 mg.

HATO MUGI

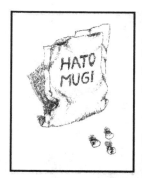

Hato mugi (also known as *pearl barley* and *Job's tears*) is a grain that is smaller, whiter, and more compact than ordinary barley. In addition to its nutritional value, it is prized as a beauty aid and as a medicinal food.

Varieties & Use: Hato mugi is available at selected natural foods stores and from macrobiotic mail-order companies. A concentrated form, *hato mugi malt*, is used as a sweetener. *Hato mugi tea* is available in tea bags. Pearl barley should not be confused with pearled barley, a form of polished barley. Hato mugi **is** prepared as a small side dish, cooked with brown rice or other grain, or added to soups and stews.

Health Benefits: Hato mugi melts excess animal protein and fat and beautifies the skin. As an external remedy, a *pearl barley plaster* is good for harmonizing body energy and drawing out and softening excess fat or protein. It is especially good for clearing up moles, warts, and boils.

Recipe for Brown Rice with Hato Mugi: Soak 1 1/2 cups of brown rice and 1/2 cup hato mugi 6-8 hours and pressure cook with 3 cups spring water, adding a pinch of salt as pot comes up to pressure. Cook for 50 minutes and garnish with parsley.

Cost: $4.75/lb.; Premium $12.00/lb.; year-round

Composition of Hato Mugi, 100 Grams, Edible Portion

Water 13.0 gm.	Calories 375	Protein 14.2 gm.	Fat 5.9 gm.	Carbo. 64.8 gm.	Fiber 0.8 gm.	Calcium 11 mg.	Phos. 300 mg.
Iron 2.5 mg.	Sodium 1 mg.	Potass. 320 mg.	Vit. A 0	Thiamin 0.27 mg	Ribofla. 0.11 mg.	Niacin 1.3 mg.	Vit. C 0

HIZIKI

Hiziki (also spelled *hijiki*) is a brown, pine-needle-shaped sea vegetable that turns black when cooked. It grows in East Asian seas. Harvested in the spring and dried, hijiki has a strong flavor of the sea when cooked and is popular for its nutty aroma.

Varieties & Use: Hiziki is enjoyed as a small side dish sautéed kinpira style. It goes well with root vegetables, deep-fried or dried tofu, or tempeh. Hizjiki rolls, made with sliced vegetables and tofu in a whole wheat pie crust and baked, are very tasty. With vegetables, it makes a refreshing salad.

Health Benefits: Hiziki has one of the highest concentrations of calcium and iron of any foods and is an excellent source of minerals and trace elements, as well as vitamins A, C, and B_{12}. It helps reduce serum cholesterol and prevents heart disease.

Recipe for Hiziki with Onions: Wash and drain 1 oz. of hiziki. Sauté 2 onions, sliced, for 2-3 minutes in 1 tsp. dark sesame oil. Put the hiziki on top, add spring water to cover just the onions, bring to a boil, lower heat, and add 1 Tbsp. of shoyu. Cover, simmer for 45-60 minutes, add 1 Tbsp. of shoyu or to taste, simmer for another 15-20 minutes or until liquid evaporates.

Cost: $5.00-7.00/1.76-2 oz.; year-round

Composition of Hiziki, 100 Grams, Edible Portion

Water 13.6 gm.	Calories --	Protein 10.6 gm.	Fat 1.3 gm.	Carbo. 47.0 gm.	Fiber 9.2 gm.	Calcium 1400 mg	Phos. 100 mg.
Iron 55 mg.	Sodium 1400 mg	Potass. 4400 mg	Vit. A 310 I.U.	Thiamin 0.01 mg.	Ribofla. 0.14 mg.	Niacin 1.8 mg.	Vit. C 0

KALE

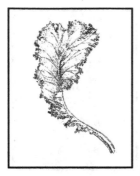

Kale is a dark, leafy green vegetable with tight, curly leaves and a hard, fibrous stalk. It has a full, sweet taste, cooks up very tender, and gives strong energy.

Varieties & Use: Usually available year round, the winter variety that survives under snow and ice and is harvested in early spring is the most tender and hardy. Kale may be boiled, steamed, or sautéed. Kale is often served with an umeboshi vinegar sauce, a tofu dressing, a lemon sauce, or a miso sauce.

Health Benefits: Kale's upward energy is beneficial to the liver and gallbladder. An excellent source of calcium and iron, kale creates strong bones and teeth and helps prevent osteoporosis. It is also high in vitamins A and C. Made into leafy greens juice, it helps dissolve heavy, stagnant protein, fat, and cholesterol deposits and relieve liver disorders. Chopped and mashed into a *chlorophyll plaster*, it is good for cooling down fever or neutralizing inflammation.

Recipe for Steamed Kale: Steam 4 cups washed and thinly sliced kale in a little water for a few minutes. The kale should be bright green and slightly crisp.

Cost: $1.50-2.00/lb.; peak winter

Composition of Kale, 100 Grams, Edible Portion

Water	Calories	Protein	Fat	Carbo.	Fiber	Calcium	Phos.
84.5 gm.	50	3.3 gm.	0.7 gm.	10.0 gm.	2.0 gm.	135 mg.	56 mg.
Iron	Sodium	Potass.	Vit. A	Thiamin	Ribofla.	Niacin	Vit. C
1.7 mg.	43 mg.	447 mg.	8900 IU.	0.11 mg	0.13 mg.	1.0 mg.	120 mg.

KOMBU

Kombu, a large, thick sea vegetable of the kelp family, cooks up dark green and has a mild taste and firm texture.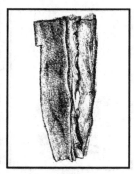

Varieties & Use: The Japanese variety, with wide, thick fronds, is gathered off Hokkaido. It is also available as strands (*natto kombu*) and in finely shaven, paper thin strips soaked in brown rice vinegar (*tororo kombu*). Kombu is used to make *dashi*, the broth used as a stock for soup and noodle dishes. It is also prepared as a side dish, cooked with grains, beans, or root vegetables, and made into condiments, pickles, and teas.

Health Benefits: The subject of widespread medical research, kombu strengthens the blood, eliminates toxic wastes (including radioactivity) from the body, and as a food or compress can help prevent and reduce tumors, especially those of the breast.

Recipe for Boiled Kombu and Vegetables: Wash and soak 1 strip of kombu, 10-12 inches long, for 3-5 min. Slice in half, cut in 1-inch pieces, and put in a pot. Add 1 onion, peeled and quartered, 1 carrot cut into triangular shapes, and soaking water to half cover the vegetables. Bring to a boil, reduce heat, simmer for 30 min. Add 1 tsp. shoyu and cook for 10 more min.

Cost: $5.00-6.00/1.76-2 oz.; year-round

Composition of Kombu, 100 Grams, Edible Portion

Water	Calories	Protein	Fat	Carbo.	Fiber	Calcium	Phos.
12.3 gm.	--	7.9 gm.	0.5 gm.	49.3 gm.	5.3 gm.	680 mg.	250 mg.
Iron	Sodium	Potass.	Vit. A	Thiamin	Ribofla.	Niacin	Vit. C
3.3 mg.	3100 mg	7500 mg	240 I.U.	0.21 mg.	0.32 mg.	1.5 mg.	0

KUZU

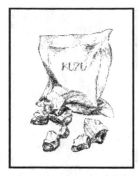

Kuzu (also known as *kudzu*) comes from the deep roots of a wild vine and is traditionally used as a thickener for sauces, gravies, puddings, and other dishes.

Varieties & Use: Japanese kuzu is available in powdered form in natural foods stores and from macrobiotic mail order companies. It grows wild throughout the South. Avoid the kuzu in Oriental markets that includes potato starch or white rice powder. Kuzu can substitute for cornstarch, egg whites, and other thickeners in cooking.

Health Benefits: Kuzu gives calm, balanced energy. It stabilizes body temperature and metabolism. Its soothing and neutralizing properties make it the base for many home remedies such as *ume-sho kuzu drink* to promote digestion and restore energy.

Recipe for Ume-Sho Kuzu Drink: Dissolve 1 tsp. of kuzu in 2-3 Tbsp. of cold water. Add 1 cup cold water, 1/2-1 umeboshi plum chopped and ground into a paste. Bring to a boil, stirring constantly to avoid lumping, until translucent. Add several drops shoyu, stirring gently, and simmer 2-3 minutes. Drink hot.

Cost: Powder $5.00/4 oz.; $18.00/lb. ; year-round

Composition of Kuzu, 100 Grams, Edible Portion

Water	Calories	Protein	Fat	Carbo.	Fiber	Calcium	Phos.
13.9 gm.	347	0.2 gm.	0.2 gm.	85.6 gm.	0	0.1 mg.	18 mg.
Iron	Sodium	Potass.	Vit. A	Thiamin	Ribofla.	Niacin	Vit. C
2.0 mg.	2 mg.	2 mg.	0	0	0	0	0

LENTILS

Lentils are a traditional staple in the Middle East, Southern Europe, India, and parts of South and Southeast Asia.

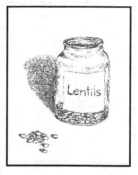

Varieties & Use: *Green lentils,* the Middle Eastern type, is green to brown in color and *red lentils,* the Indian variety, is orange to red. There are also *baby lentils,* which are much smaller and finer than usual lentils. Lentils make a nourishing soup by itself or cooked with barley or other grain. They are also enjoyed prepared with carrots, onions, celery, winter squash, and other ingredients. Burdock gives lentils a strong taste and energy. In India they are curried to make *dhal* which is eaten with rice.

Health Benefits: High in nutrients, lentils are the main source of protein in many cultures. They are also high in calcium, iron, complex carbohydrates, and dietary fiber, which are strengthening to digestion, circulation, and the nervous system.

Recipe for Lentil Soup: Layer 2 onions, diced, 1 carrot, diced, and 1 cup of dried and washed lentils in a pot. Add 1 qt. of spring water and pinch of sea salt. Bring to a boil, reduce heat, cover, and simmer for 45 min. Add 1 Tbsp. of chopped parsley and more salt to taste. Simmer for 20 min. longer and serve.

Cost: Green Lentils $.75-1.00/lb.; year-round

Composition of Lentils, 100 Grams, Edible Portion

Water	Calories	Protein	Fat	Carbo.	Fiber	Calcium	Phos.
80.1 gm.	72	1.5 gm.	0.2 gm.	17.4 gm.	3.3 gm.	47 mg.	71 mg.
Iron	Sodium	Potass.	Vit. A	Thiamin	Ribofla.	Niacin	Vit. C
0.8 mg.	5.0 mg.	308 mg.	0 I.U.	0.01 mg.	0.03 mg.	0.3 mg.	3 mg.

LOTUS ROOT

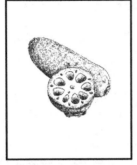

Lotus, the long, chambered root of the lotus plant, is enjoyed for its creamy-white color, firm, crisp texture, and mild taste.

Varieties & Use: Fresh lotus root is enjoyed sautéed with other root vegetables such as burdock or carrots or sea vegetables such as arame or hijiki; boiled *nishime* style with shiitake and daikon; or in marinades. It is also delicious tempura style, deep-fried, or stuffed with miso or tahini. *Dried lotus root* and *dried* or *powdered lotus root tea* are also available. *Lotus seeds,* from the same plant, may be added to rice, beans or vegetables.

Health Benefits: Lotus root helps to dissolve mucus and fat in the lungs, bronchi, throat, and sinuses, especially from dairy food or egg consumption. *Lotus root tea* helps relieve lung congestion, clear up sinus problems, and ease chronic coughing. A *lotus root plaster* helps disperse and remove stagnated mucus in the respiratory system.

Recipe for Sautéed Lotus Root: Slice 1 cup onions in half moons and sauté for several minutes. Add 1/4 cup spring water, layer 2 cups sliced lotus root on top of the onions, cover, and bring to a boil. Reduce flame and simmer 3-5 min. more.

Cost: Fresh $4.00/lb.; Dried $5.00/1.76-2 oz.; year-round

Composition of Lotus Root, 100 Grams, Edible Portion

Water	Calories	Protein	Fat	Carbo.	Fiber	Calcium	Phos.
79.1 gm.	74	2.6 gm.	0.1 gm.	17.2 gm.	4.9 gm.	45 mg.	100 mg.
Iron	Sodium	Potass.	Vit. A	Thiamin	Ribofla.	Niacin	Vit. C
1.2 mg.	40 mg	556 mg.	0	0.16 mg.	0.22 mg.	0.4 mg.	44 mg.

MILLET

This nutritious, small, compact whole grain has been traditionally eaten in China, Africa, and southern Europe, especially Italy.

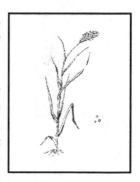

Varieties & Use: Yellow millet is available in the West, while red varieties predominate in the East. Millet fluffs up when cooked and makes a light, attractive dish. It is often served with a miso sauce, kuzu-ginger gravy, or other topping. Millet-rice, made by cooking 20% millet with 80% brown rice, is stronger and sweeter than regular brown rice. Millet also goes well with cauliflower, winter squash, azuki beans, or lentils and can be used in croquettes and stuffings. Millet can also be dry-roasted, baked, or pounded and shaped into loaves or cakes.

Health Benefits: Millet gives strong, harmonious energy. It nourishes the pancreas, spleen, and stomach and is especially recommended for diabetes, hypoglycemia, lymphoma, and other disorders associated with these organs. Millet contributes to practical, creative thinking and sympathy with others.

Recipe for Soft Millet: Wash 1 cup of millet, place in pot, and add 3 cups of spring water. Bring to a boil, add pinch of sea salt, cover, and cook 30 min. Serve as a delicious porridge.

Cost: $.65-75 lb.; year-round

Composition of Millet, 100 Grams, Edible Portion

Water	Calories	Protein	Fat	Carbo.	Fiber	Calcium	Phos.
8.7 gm.	378	11.0 gm.	4.2 gm.	72.9 gm.	8.5 gm.	8.0 mg.	285 mg.
Iron	Sodium	Potass.	Vit. A	Thiamin	Ribofla.	Niacin	Vit. E
3.0 mg.	5.0 mg	195 mg.	0	0.42 mg.	0.29 mg.	4.7 mg.	0.18 mg.

MISO

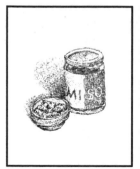

Miso is a nourishing, mildly sweet-tasting paste or purée made from soybeans, sea salt, and usually fermented barley or brown rice. A staple of Far Eastern cooking, miso soup and other dishes seasoned with miso have spread around the world.

Varieties & Use: Principal types include barley (*mugi*) miso, 100% soybean (*hatcho*), and brown rice (*genmai*), and those aged two years or more are the standard for daily macrobiotic cooking. Sweet misos (*red, yellow,* or *white*), aged 6 months, are used for sauces and special dishes. *Instant miso* is available for traveling. Besides soups, miso is used in pickling, marinades, preparing sauces, spreads, and dressings, and seasoning other dishes.

Health Benefits: Miso contains enzymes that facilitate digestion and strengthens blood quality. High in protein, B vitamins, and minerals, miso helps relieve breast cancer, heart disease, and radiation sickness. It is used as a plaster for cuts and burns.

Recipe for Miso Soup: Place a 3-inch piece of rinsed wakame, sliced into 1/2-inch pieces, 1 cup sliced onions, and 1 qt. water in a pot. Bring to a boil, lower heat, simmer for 4-5 min. Add 1 Tbsp. miso, simmer for 3-5 min., and garnish with scallions.

Cost: Two-Year Barley $3.50/8 oz.; $6.00-8.00/lb.; year-round

Composition of Barley Miso, 100 Grams, Edible Portion

Water	Calories	Protein	Fat	Carbo.	Fiber	Calcium	Phos.
44.0 gm.	198	9.7 gm.	4.3 gm.	28.3 gm.	1.7 gm.	80 mg.	120 mg.
Iron	Sodium	Potass.	Vit. A	Thiamin	Ribofla.	Niacin	Vit. C
3.0 mg.	4200 mg	340 mg.	0	0.04 mg.	0.10 mg.	1.5 mg.	0

MOCHI

Delicious dumplings, cubes, or cakes made from pounded sweet rice are known as mochi. A traditional New Year's treat in Japan, mochi is now part of a planetary cuisine. It is especially enjoyed as a snack or dessert by women and children.

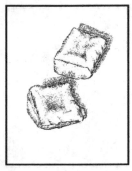

Varieties & Use: Mochi can be made at home or be obtained ready-made (plain, with mugwort, or spiced). Cut into many shapes and sizes, it is enjoyed pan fried (with oil or plain), steamed, boiled, or baked. In casseroles, mochi strips may be added on top for a melted cheese-like effect. Mochi puffs up when cooked and produces scrumptious waffles.

Health Benefits: Mochi provides warmth and energy. It is given to pregnant or lactating mothers or anyone needing strength and vitality. It also helps increase weight. Mochi's sweet taste nourishes the pancreas, spleen, and stomach.

Recipe for Pan Fried Mochi: Place 1-inch squares of mochi in a dry, heated skillet. Cover, cook over low heat for 2-3 min. Turn mochi over, cook another few minutes until they begin to puff up. Enjoy plain or topped with barley malt, shoyu, or natural preserves.

Cost: $2.50-4.00/12 oz. package; Japanese import $6.50/8.8 oz.

Composition of Mochi, 100 Grams, Edible Portion

Water	Calories	Protein	Fat	Carbo.	Fiber	Calcium	Phos.
44.5 gm.	235	4.2 gm.	0.8 gm.	50.1 gm.	0.2 gm.	3 mg.	50 mg.
Iron	Sodium	Potass.	Vit. A	Thiamin	Ribofla.	Niacin	Vit. C
0.1 mg.	2 mg.	43 mg.	0	0.06 mg.	0.02 mg.	0.6 mg.	0

MUSTARD GREENS

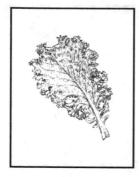

Mustard greens have crisp, delicate leaves, a pungent, sweet taste, and give strong, hearty energy.

Varieties & Use: Growing through the winter, the mustard plant blooms in the spring and reaches a peak between December and March. Mustard seed oil, processed from this plant, yields a high-quality cooking oil. *Yellow mustard* is made from the same plant. Mustard greens may be lightly boiled, steamed, or sautéed and served as a small side dish. They go well with onions.

Health Benefits: Like other leafy green vegetables high in calcium, mustard greens are excellent for maintaining bone density and preventing osteoporosis. They are also loaded with vitamin A and high in thiamin, riboflavin, and vitamin C. Energetically, they are especially good for the heart and small intestine. They may be used medicinally in leafy greens juice or externally as a *chlorophyll plaster*.

Recipe for Mustard Greens with a Shoyu-Ginger Sauce: Boil 4 cups thinly sliced mustard greens in 1/4-inch of spring water for several minutes, keeping bright and crisp. Mix 1/4 cup shoyu, 1/4 cup water, and 1/2 tsp. grated ginger for sauce.

Cost: $1.50-2.00/lb.; peak winter

Composition of Mustard Greens, 100 Grams, Edible Portion

Water	Calories	Protein	Fat	Carbo.	Fiber	Calcium	Phos.
90.8 gm.	26	2.7 gm.	0.2 gm.	4.9 gm.	3.3 gm.	103 mg.	43 mg.
Iron	Sodium	Potass.	Vit. A	Thiamin	Ribofla.	Niacin	Vit. C
1.5 mg.	25 mg.	354 mg.	5300 IU.	0.08 mg.	0.11 mg.	0.8 mg.	70 mg.

NATTO

Natto, a fermented soybean product that has been steamed and partially mashed, resembles baked beans connected by long, sticky strands. Its funky odor puts off some people, while many others appreciate its delicious taste, mucilaginous texture, and strong aroma.

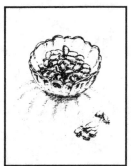

Varieties & Use: Natto can be made at home or be purchased in frozen form in the natural foods store or from mail order suppliers. Natto is enjoyed warmed up as a small side dish or condiment for brown rice, soba, or mochi. It is customarily served with shoyu, scallions, chives, mustard, grated ginger, grated dakon, horseradish, or other seasoning or garnishes. It may also be sautéed or deep-fried, and natto sushi is very tasty.

Health Benefits: Natto is very beneficial to digestion and strengthens the intestines, blood, lymph, and kidneys.

Recipe for Natto with Scallions: Mash 1/2 cup natto in a mortar with mustard to taste. Mix in chopped scallions and serve.

Cost: Frozen container, $3.00/5-oz.

Composition of Natto, 100 Grams, Edible Portion

Water	Calories	Protein	Fat	Carbo.	Fiber	Calcium	Phos.
55.0 gm.	212	17.7 gm.	11.0 gm.	14.4 gm.	5.4 gm.	217 mg.	174 mg.
Iron	Sodium	Potass.	Vit. A	Thiamin	Ribofla.	Niacin	Vit. C
8.6 mg.	7.0 mg.	729 mg.	0	0.16 mg.	0.19 mg.	0	13 mg.

NOODLES

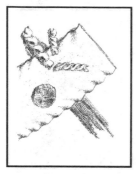

Nearly everyone enjoys noodles and pasta. Noodles made with whole grain flour and other high quality ingredients are now unifying East and West and make a delicious meal or convenient snack.

Varieties & Use: Far Eastern style noodles include *udon* (whole wheat), *somen* (thin whole wheat), *ramen* (pre-steamed or fried whole wheat), *bifun* (rice), and *soba* (from 40-100% buckwheat and whole wheat). Western types include *whole wheat spaghetti, linguini, lasagna, angel hair, spirals, elbows,* and others. Noodles are enjoyed plain in broth or served with vegetables, tofu or tempeh, sea vegetables, or other ingredients. They may be boiled, fried, baked, or made *nabe* style.

Health Benefits: Noodles give quick, warming energy and often have a rich, satisfying taste.

Recipe for Noodles in Broth: Bring 6-8 cups of spring water to boil, add 8-oz. of udon, return to a boil, and cook for 10 minutes. When done, rinse in cold water to prevent clumping, serve with a broth made of a small piece of kombu, 2 dried shiitakes, and 2 Tbsp. shoyu cooked together for 3-5 minutes. Garnish with scallions, chives, or toasted nori.

Cost: Udon $2.50-3.00/7-8 oz.; $5.00/lb.; year round

Composition of Udon, 100 Grams, Edible Portion

Water	Calories	Protein	Fat	Carbo.	Fiber	Calcium	Phos.
76.5 gm.	101	2.5 gm.	0.5 gm.	20.3 gm.	0.1 gm.	7 mg.	18 mg.
Iron	Sodium	Potass.	Vit. A	Thiamin	Ribofla.	Niacin	Vit. C
0.2 mg.	45 mg.	6 mg.	0	0.02 mg.	0.01 mg.	0.1 mg.	0

NORI

Nori (also known as *laver*) is best known as the thin, dark green sea vegetable used to wrap sushi rolls and rice balls.

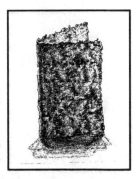

Varieties & Use: Nori is available in wafer-thin sheets, in flakes and strips, and mixed in a variety of snack foods. Most nori is harvested in Japan, but laver from off the Maine seacoast is also available. In addition to sushi and rice balls, nori is used as a garnish for salads, soups, noodles, rice, or casseroles. Nori condiment is made by cooking into a thick paste with shoyu.

Health Benefits: Nori is rich in nutrients, including protein, calcium, iron, vitamin A, and vitamin C. It is especially beneficial for the kidneys and urinary function, reproductive organs, and like other sea vegetables helps reduce cholesterol and improve circulation, offset tumor development, and protect against radiation. It is added to *carrot-daikon drink.*

Recipe for Toasted Nori: Toast a sheet of nori over the burner by holding the shiny side about 6 inches over low heat and twirling for 15-30 seconds until the sheet turns from purple to green. Enjoy as a snack or use as a garnish for other dishes.

Cost: 10 Sheets $6.00; 50 sheets $27.00; year-round

Composition of Nori, 100 Grams, Edible Portion

Water 11.1 gm.	Calories --	Protein 38.8 gm.	Fat 1.9 gm.	Carbo. 39.5 gm.	Fiber 1.8 gm.	Calcium 390 mg.	Phos. 580 mg.
Iron 12 mg.	Sodium 120 mg.	Potass. 2100 mg	Vit. A 14000	Thiamin 1.15 mg	Ribofla. 3.4 mg.	Niacin 9.8 mg.	Vit. C 100 mg.

OATS

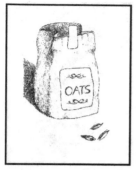

Oats are tasty and give strong, hardy energy. Hailing from Northern Europe, especially Scotland and Ireland, they are now grown around the world and softly prepared make a popular morning porridge.

Varieties & Use: *Whole oats*, from which only the outer husks have been removed, provide the most energy and vitality. *Scotch oats* have been steamed and steel-cut into smaller pieces. *Rolled oats* (common *oatmeal*) have been steamed and passed through rollers. Oats are also available processed into flakes, puffed oats, and flour. Oats are enjoyed plain or mixed with grains, added to soups, stews, or casseroles. *Rolled oats* or *oat flour* are often added to breads, cookies, puddings, and granola and make chewy desserts and baked goods.

Health Benefits: Oats have more fat than other grains, give a warm energy, and provide stamina and endurance. They are particular strengthening for the the liver and gallbladder.

Recipe for Whole Oatmeal: Wash 1 cup whole oats, soak for several hours or overnight, place in a pot. Add 5-6 cups spring water, pinch of sea salt, cover, and bring to a boil. Reduce heat, simmer over low heat for several hours until water is absorbed.

Cost: Whole Oats $.75-1.00/lb.; year round

Composition of Oats, 100 Grams, Edible Portion

Water 8.2 gm.	Calories 389	Protein 16.9 gm.	Fat 6.9 gm.	Carbo. 66.3 gm.	Fiber 10.6 gm.	Calcium 54 mg.	Phos. 523 mg.
Iron 4.7 mg.	Sodium 2.0 mg.	Potass. 429 mg.	Vit. A 0	Thiamin 0.76 mg.	Ribofla. 0.14 mg.	Niacin 1.0 mg.	Vit. E 0.7 mg.

ONION

Onions have a pleasant, round shape; pungent flavor and odor; juicy, many-layered bulb; and a sweet taste that combines well with many other foods and dishes.

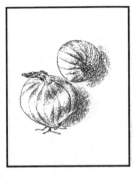

Varieties & Use: Onions come in many shapes, sizes, and colors. Popular varieties include *Bermuda onion* (mild white or yellow), *Spanish onion* (large yellow or white), *Italian onion* (red), *Vidalia* (large, pale onions from Georgia), and *pearl onions* (tiny, mild, and creamy when cooked). Onions are enjoyed in salads, soups, stir-fries, marinades, and pickles.

Health Benefits: Cooked onions give a calm, peaceful energy. They are especially soothing for nervous conditions, for muscle aches and pains, and when cooked with squash and carrots as a sweet dish for diabetic conditions. Raw onion is traditionally taken on an empty stomach as a treatment for worms.

Recipe for Whole Onions and Miso: Place 6 whole onions, partially cut, in a pot with a long strip of soaked kombu. Add water to half cover. Pour 1 Tbsp. puréed miso on top, cover, bring to a boil. Lower heat and simmer 30 min. or until soft.

Cost: $.75-1.25/lb.; peak autumn-winter

Composition of Onion, 100 Grams, Edible Portion

Water	Calories	Protein	Fat	Carbo.	Fiber	Calcium	Phos.
89.7 gm.	38	1.2 gm.	0.2 gm.	8.6 gm.	1.8 gm.	20 mg.	33 mg.
Iron	Sodium	Potass.	Vit. A	Thiamin	Ribofla.	Niacin	Vit. C
0.2 mg.	3 mg.	157 mg.	0	0.04 mg.	0.02 mg.	0.2 mg.	6. 4 mg.

PARSLEY

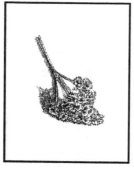

Parsley has a bright green color, soft texture, and mildly sharp taste that make it a nutritious side dish or addition to grain and vegtetable dishes, as well as a popular garnish and flavoring.

Varieties & Use: Parsley comes in bunches at the marketplace. Popular varieties include *curly-leaf parsley* and *flat-leaf* or *Italian parlsey* which has a stronger flavor. Parsley may be added to soups, salads, and grain and vegetable dishes. It combines especially well with yellow or orange foods such as millet, squash, and corn. Dipped in boiling water for only a few seconds, parsley's bright green color turns even deeper. The stems are fibrous and may be boiled or sautéed slightly longer.

Health Benefits: Parlsey is loaded with calcium and iron and has one of the highest concentrations of vitamin A of any food. It is also high in fiber, B vitamins, and vitamin C.

Recipe for Parsley with Ginger Sauce: Boil 1 bunch parsley in 1/4 inch of spring water and a pinch of sea salt. Cook for a few seconds, remove, and let cool. Combine 1 tsp. shoyu, 1/4 tsp. grated fresh ginger, and a little parsley water for sauce. Chop parlsley, add sauce, and garnish with sesame seeds.

Cost: $.75-1.00/lb.; peak summer-autumn

Composition of Parsley, 100 Grams, Edible Portion

Water 87.7 gm.	Calories 36	Protein 3.0 gm.	Fat 0.8 gm.	Carbo. 6.3 gm.	Fiber 3.3 gm.	Calcium 138 mg.	Phos. 58 mg.
Iron 6.2 mg.	Sodium 56 mg.	Potass. 554 mg.	Vit. A 5200 IU.	Thiamin 0.09 mg	Riboffa. 0.10 mg.	Niacin 1.3 mg.	Vit. C 133 mg.

PARSNIP

Parsnips originated in Europe and have a beautiful, smooth white color, soft, crisp texture, and sweet, succulent taste.

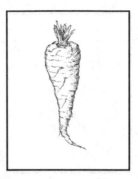

Varieties & Use: Parsnips are often prepared as a side dish. They also combine well with other foods, especially carrots and onions, and may be served with a sauce made from clear soup stock, kuzu root, and grated ginger. Parsnips may be boiled, steamed, sautéed, deep-fried, pickled, or prepared tempura style. In macrobiotic cooking, they are frequently mashed and turned into a pie crust or cake and are surprisingly sweet. They may also be fried into chips.

Health Benefits: Parnsips have a balance of nutrients and energy that contribute to health at many levels. Their sweet taste is especially beneficial to the pancreas, spleen, and stomach.

Recipe for Parsnip Cake: Bring 2 cups apple juice and a pinch of sea salt to a boil. Add 1 cup couscous, turn off heat, and let the couscous absorb the liquid. Place in a cake pan. Separately, cook 1 pound parsnips with 1 cup apple juice and a pinch of sea salt. After about 10 minutes, when the parsnips are soft, purée in a food mill, spread parsnips on the couscous, and serve.

Cost: $1.00/lb.; peak autumn-winter

Composition of Parsnip, 100 Grams, Edible Portion

Water	Calories	Protein	Fat	Carbo.	Fiber	Calcium	Phos.
79.5 gm.	75	1.2 gm.	0.3 gm.	18.0 gm.	4.9 gm.	36 mg.	71 mg.
Iron	Sodium	Potass.	Vit. A	Thiamin	Ribofla.	Niacin	Vit. C
0.6 mg.	10 mg.	375 mg.	0	0.09 mg.	0.05 mg.	0.7mg.	17 mg.

RADISH

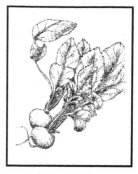

Radishes come in a variety of colors, shapes, and flavors and are enjoyed in salads, as pickles, and as a garnish.

Varieties & Use: *Red radishes* are most common, while *white, purple,* and *black radishes* are selectively available. (See *Daikon* for the large Oriental style radish.) Radishes may be round, oval, or elongated. *Radish tops* may be cooked and served as a small side dish, and *radish sprouts* are nice in salads. The pungent taste of radish makes them popular raw, lightly boiled, or pressed in salads. Radish and radish tops are traditionally pickled with umeboshi plums.

Health Benefits: Radishes have a balance of nutrients and energy. They are high in calcium and vitamin C. Energetically, radishes are beneficial for the lungs and large intestine. Though not as strong as daikon, red radish may be substituted in medicinal teas or as a plaster for bruises and inflammations.

Recipe for Red Radishes and Kuzu Sauce: Place 10 whole radishes, tops removed, in a pot with a small piece of kombu and 1-2 umeboshi plums. Cook 30-40 min. over low heat. Remove radishes, and thicken liquid with 1-2 tsp. diluted kuzu.

Cost: $.75-1.00/lb.; peak spring-summer

Composition of Radish, 100 Grams, Edible Portion

Water	Calories	Protein	Fat	Carbo.	Fiber	Calcium	Phos.
94.8 gm.	20	0.6 gm.	0.5 gm.	3.6 gm.	1.6 gm.	21 mg.	18 mg.
Iron	Sodium	Potass.	Vit. A	Thiamin	Ribofla.	Niacin	Vit. C
0.3 mg.	24 mg.	232 mg.	8 IU.	0.01 mg	0.05 mg.	0.3 mg.	22.8 mg.

RYE

Rye, a traditional whole grain in Russia, Scandinavia, and other northern areas, gives hardy energy. It is best known for producing delightfully chewy, dark bread.

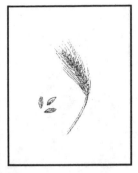

Varieties & Use: *Whole rye, rye flour, rye flakes,* and other rye products are available in natural foods stores. Rye is harder than other grains and requires soaking for several hours or overnight. In whole form, it is usually cooked with other grains (e.g., 20% rye and 80% brown rice) and produces an enjoyable, chewy dish. Rye may also be cooked together with carrots, onions, and other vegetables. Rye flour is added to whole wheat flour to make rye bread, crackers, and other baked products.

Health Benefits: Rye is high in protein, calcium, iron, B vitamins, and other nutrients. It gives energy and vitality and is especially beneficial to respiratory and excretory functions.

Recipe for Brown Rice with Rye: Pressure cook 1/2 cup of rye and 1 1/2 cups of brown rice together in 3 cups of spring water and a pinch or two of sea salt for 50 minutes. Soak or dry-roast rye beforehand to make it more digestible.

Cost: $1.00-1.50; year round

Composition of Rye, 100 Grams, Edible Portion

Water	Calories	Protein	Fat	Carbo.	Fiber	Calcium	Phos.
11.0 gm.	335	14.8 gm.	2.5 gm.	69.8 gm.	14.6 gm.	33 mg.	374 mg.
Iron	Sodium	Potass.	Vit. A	Thiamin	Ribofla.	Niacin	Vit. E
2.7 mg.	6 mg.	264 mg.	0	0.32 mg.	0.25 mg.	4.3 mg.	1.9 mg.

SCALLION

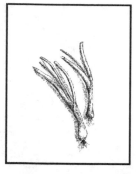

Scallion's small white bulb and bright, long green leaves give it a unique shape, energy, and taste. This versatile vegetable is enjoyed in salads and as a garnish.

Varieties & Use: Scallions are widely available and easy to grow in the garden. As a garnish, scallions combine well with grains, noodles, soups, stews, beans, tofu, tempeh, natto, and vegetables. They may be used raw or be boiled or sautéed for a few seconds. Scallions are traditionally prepared into a sweet condiment with miso. The tiny white roots of the scallion are very high in nutrients and energy and may be chopped and used in cooking.

Health Benefits: Scallions stimulate the appetite and senses. They are high in calcium, vitamin A, vitamin C, and other nutrients. They give warm energy and are especially strengthening for the liver and gallbladder.

Recipe for Scallion-Miso Condiment: Wash 2-3 bunches of scallions and roots. Place in a skillet oiled with 1 Tbsp. sesame oil. Form a hollow in the scallions and pour 3 tsp. puréed miso into center. Cover, simmer for 5 minutes, mix, and serve.

Cost: $.75-1.00/bunch; year-round

Composition of Scallion, 100 Grams, Edible Portion

Water 89.4 gm.	Calories 36	Protein 1.5 gm.	Fat 0.2 gm.	Carbo. 8.2 gm.	Fiber 1.2 gm.	Calcium 66 mg.	Phos. 39 mg.
Iron 0.4 mg.	Sodium 5 mg.	Potass. 239 mg.	Vit. A 580 I.U.	Thiamin 0.07 mg	Ribofla. 0.07 mg.	Niacin 1.1 mg.	Vit. C 43 mg.

SEA SALT

Salt is essential to life and one of humanity's oldest staples. *Unrefined sea salt* (evaporated from the ocean) preserves many of the minerals and trace elements refined from ordinary table salt.

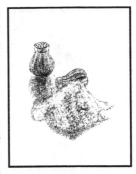

Varieties & Use: *White sea salt* flows freely, and tastes slightly sweet and then gradually turns salty. It is preferred for daily use. *Grey sea salt* may be used externally. Salt is added to whole grains, beans, vegetables, and other foods during cooking rather than at the table. A small pinch of salt may be added to cooked or fresh fruit to give a sweet taste. Salt is used in pickling, marinades, and dry-roasted to make *gomashio.*

Health Benefits: Human blood corresponds with the ancient ocean in which life began. Salt is essential to strong blood, lymph, and bodily fluids, as well as digestion and nervous functioning. Sea salt is beneficial to the kidneys, bladder, heart, and small intestine. A *salt pack* reduces inflammation.

Recipe for Chinese Cabbage Pickles: Place 2 cups of thinly sliced Chinese cabbage in a pickle press or bowl with a saucer and weight. Sprinkle 1-2 tsp. of sea salt and mix with the cabbage. Press for several hours and rinse pickles before serving.

Cost: $2.00-3.00/pound; year-round

Composition of Sea Salt vs. Table Salt

Sea Salt	NaCL 97.51%	Mg Carb. 1.51%	Ca Chl. 0.40%	Pot. Sul. 0.42%	Fl, St, Br 0.14%	Trace Elements 0.003%
Table Salt	NaCL 99.5%	Magnesium carbonate, potassium iodide, dextrose (sugar), sodium carbonate 0.5% *Source: East West Jurnal, 1983*				

SEITAN

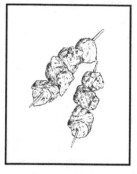

Seitan (also known as *wheat meat*) is a dynamic, rich-tasting food made from wheat gluten cooked with shoyu and kombu. It is popular in veggie burgers, stir-fries, cutlets, and other dishes.

Varieties & Use: Seitan can be made at home or be purchased fresh at the natural foods store. A small bottled form of seitan imported from Japan is also available. *Fu* is a softer form of wheat gluten that has been steamed and dehydrated. Seitan is frequently cooked *kinpira* style with burdock, carrots, and celery; sautéed with onions; boiled with sauerkraut; deep-fried with root vegetables; made into croquettes; pan-fried into burgers; or added to soups, stews, and salads.

Health Benefits: High in protein, calcium, iron, and other minerals, seitan gives strength, energy, and contributes to general good health. As part of a balanced diet, it is strengthening to the liver and gallbladder.

Recipe for Sautéed Seitan and Onions: Sauté 2 cups sliced onions, topped with 2 cups sliced seitan, in 2 Tbsp. dark sesame oil. Cover, simmer 10 minutes or until onions are translucent. Mix and simmer 3-5 minutes. Garnish with parsley and serve.

Cost: $3.00/8-ounce package; year-round

Composition of Seitan, 100 Grams, Edible Portion

Water	Calories	Protein	Fat	Carbo.	Fiber	Calcium	Phos.
--	118	18.0 gm.	--	--	0.1 gm.	19 mg.	44 mg.
Iron	Sodium	Potass.	Vit. A	Thiamin	Ribofla.	Niacin	Vit. C
3.6 mg.	--	38 mg.	0	0.03 mg	0.02 mg.	0.8 mg.	0

SESAME SEEDS

Sesame seeds have been traditionally eaten in the Far East, Middle East, Mediterranean, Africa, and South America.

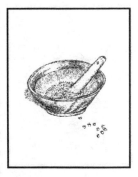

Varieties & Use: The tiny round seeds come into two main varieties: *white* or light brown and *black*. Sesame seeds are roasted and ground with sea salt into a flavorful and highly nutritious condiment called *gomashio*. Hulled sesame seeds are used in making *tahini*, a mild, sweet sesame paste and unhulled are used to make *sesame butter*. Unrefined *sesame oil*, pressed from these seeds, has a nutty aroma and flavorful taste.

Health Benefits: Sesame seeds are rich in protein, calcium, iron, and B vitamins. Sesame seed tea is good to darken the hair and treat menstrual irregularity. *Sesame-ginger oil* is good for arthritis, rheumatism, and ear or eye ailments.

Recipe for Gomashio: Use 1 part sea salt to 18 parts sesame seeds. Dry-roast salt for a few minutes until shiny and grind in a mortar until fine. Roast the rinsed, wet seeds for 5-10 minutes, pushing them back and forth with a paddle or wooden spoon to prevent burning. Add roasted seeds to ground salt and grind until 90% crushed. Store in an airtight container.

Cost: White $3.00/lb.; Black $4.50/lb.; Sesame Oil $5.00/10 oz.

Composition of Sesame Seeds, 100 Grams, Edible Portion

Water	Calories	Protein	Fat	Carbo.	Fiber	Calcium	Phos.
4.5 gm.	573	17.7 gm.	49.7 gm.	23.5 gm.	11.8 gm.	975 mg	629 mg.
Iron	Sodium	Potass.	Vit. A	Thiamin	Ribofla.	Niacin	Vit. C
14.6 mg.	11 mg.	468 m	9 I.U.	0.79 mg.	0.25 mg.	4.5 mg.	0

SHIITAKE

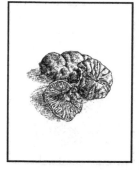

Shiitake mushrooms, a culinary and medicinal staple in the East, are now grown in the U.S. and around the world.

Varieties and Use: Fresh and dried shiitakes are available (*Donko* is the strongest variety). They are delicious boiled *nishime*-style as a side dish or as a stock for kombu broth or clear soup. Slices are commonly added to miso soup and various grain, bean, sea vegetable, and vegetable dishes. *Maitake*, another Oriental mushroom, is meatier.

Health Benefits: Shiitakes are high in protein, minerals, and B vitamins. Shiitake tea is used to reduce fever, dissolve animal fat, and help relax a contracted or tense condition. Medical studies indicate that shiitakes have an anti-tumor effect.

Recipe for Shiitake with Kombu and Dried Daikon: Wash, soak, and thinly slice 2 strips of kombu and place in a pot with 3-4 shiitakes, soaked, stemmed, and sliced. Set 1/2 cup of dried daikon, soaked and sliced on top. Add soaking water to just cover and bring to a boil. Cover, reduce heat, and simmer for 40-45 minutes or until kombu is soft. Season with shoyu to taste and simmer until remaining liquid has almost evaporated.

Cost: Fresh $11.00/lb.; Dried $7.00/1.76 oz.; year-round

Composition of Dried Shiitake, 100 Grams, Edible Portion

Water 9.5 gm.	Calories 296	Protein 9.6 gm.	Fat 1.0 gm.	Carbo. 75.4 gm.	Fiber 11.5 gm.	Calcium 11 mg.	Phos. 294 mg.
Iron 1.7 mg.	Sodium 13 mg.	Potass. 1534 mg	Vit. A 0	Thiamin 0.30 mg	Ribofla. 1.27 mg.	Niacin 14.1 mg.	Vit. C 3.5 mg.

SHOYU

Shoyu or *natural soy sauce*, a staple of Far Eastern and natural foods cooking, is used as a seasoning for soups, noodles, stir-fries, and other dishes. Its subtle flavor goes well with sweet, sour, or pungent tastes.

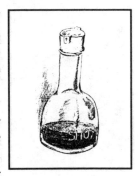

Varieties and Use: *Shoyu* is made from soybeans, wheat, sea salt, and water that have been fermented and aged in cedar vats. Commercial soy sauces are made with inferior ingredients and artificially aged. Shoyu is usually added in cooking and not at the table. It is used as a base for clear soups, a dressing or marinade for salads and quick pickles, a dipping sauce for tempura, and an ingredient in shio kombu and other condiments. *Tamari* is the liquid that rises to the top in making miso and is sold as *wheat-free tamari*. It is used sparingly, while shoyu is suitable for daily use.

Health Benefits: Shoyu aids in digesting grains and vegetables. High in protein, minerals, and B vitamins, it is used in home remedies such as *shoyu bancha tea*, which strengthens the blood, relieves fatigue, and neutralizes overacidity.

Recipe for Shoyu Bancha Tea: Place 1 tsp. of shoyu in a tea cup, pour in hot bancha twig tea, stir, and drink while hot.

Cost: $3.00/5 oz. bottle; $4.00/10 oz.; $10.00/32 oz.; year round

Composition of Shoyu, 100 Grams, Edible Portion

Water 71.1 gm.	Calories 53	Protein 5.2 gm.	Fat 0.1 gm.	Carbo. 8.5 gm.	Fiber 0.8 gm.	Calcium 17 mg.	Phos. 110 mg.
Iron 2 mg.	Sodium 5715 mg	Potass. 180 mg	Vit. A 0	Thiamin 0.05 mg.	Ribofla. 0.13 mg.	Niacin 3.4 mg.	Vit. C 0

SOYBEANS

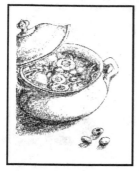

Soybeans originated in China and are now grown around the world whole or in the form of tofu, tempeh, shoyu, and other soy products. (See entries for these items.)

Varieties & Use: *Black soybeans* are stronger than *yellow soybeans* and favored for cooking and medicinal use. Black soybeans may be prepared plain or cooked with brown rice and yield a strong, delicious taste. They may also be sweetened with barley malt, rice syrup, or mirin. Black soybeans make a rich, delicious soup.

Health Benefits: Black soybeans are good for loosening, softening, and warming the body. They are made into a tea that is good for kidney, bladder, and reproductive problems caused by an accumulation of fat or excess animal food. The tea is also good for relieving dry coughs and for laryngitis. Loaded with iron and calcium, black soybeans are also good for promoting mother's milk, especially when cooked with mochi.

Recipe for Black Bean Soup: Soak 2 cups black soybeans and boil until done, about 1 1/2 -2 hours. Then purée the beans with 2-3 cups of spring water. Pour into pan, add 2 tsp. miso puréed, and simmer 3-4 minutes. Garnish with parsley or scallions.

Cost: Yellow $.75 lb.; Black $1.50/lb.; Black Hokkaido $5.00/lb.

Composition of Soybeans, 100 Grams, Edible Portion

Water 8.5 gm.	Calories 416	Protein 36.5 gm.	Fat 19.9 gm.	Carbo. 30.2 gm.	Fiber 9.3 gm.	Calcium 277 mg.	Phos. 704 mg.
Iron 15.7 mg.	Sodium 2 mg.	Potass. 1797 mg	Vit. A 24 I.U.	Thiamin 0.87 mg	Ribofla. 0.87 mg.	Niacin 1.6 mg.	Vit. C 6 mg.

SPRING WATER

Spring water is the standard for daily cooking and drinking in many macrobiotic and
natural foods households.

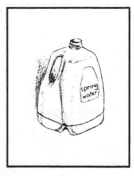

Varieties & Use: Shop around as the quality of spring waters differs widely. Preferably store in glass bottles, though plastic is
acceptable if not left unused indefinitely.
Municipal tap water usually contains cholo-
rine, fluoride, and other chemicals as well
as pesticide residues, detergents, nitrates, and heavy metals.
Distilled water lacks nutrients, is low in *Ki*, and is not recommended. *Mineral water* makes a nice party drink on occasion,
but is not suitable for regular use. If spring water is not available or too costly, *filtered tap water* is the next best alternative.
There are a wide variety of filter systems available.

Health Benefits: *Natural spring water* that is alive and moving
carries strong *Ki* or natural electromagnetic energy. Water facil-
itates digestion and absorption, balances salt and other minerals in the body, and contributes to the proper functioning of the
kidneys and bladder.

Guidelines for Drinking: Drink when thirsty, about 4 cups or
glasses a day. Modern guidelines calling for 8 or more glasses
of water are based on the consumption patterns and needs of
modern people consuming large amounts of animal quality
food. Fluid helps to offset the high sodium content and other
minerals in these foods.

Cost: $.75-1.25/gallon; $1.25-1.50/1.8 oz. bottle; year-round

Composition of Spring Water, No Standard Tables

SQUASH

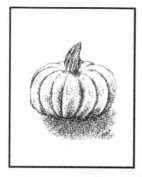

Native to North America, squashes have a deep, vibrant color; sweet, delicious taste; and make for a full, satisfying meal.

Varieties & Use: A large variety of hard winter squashes are available including *acorn, butternut, buttercup, Hokkaido, Kabocha, hubbard, delicata, spaghetti,* and *pumpkin.* They are enjoyed boiled, baked, or steamed; in soups; cooked with beans; or made into rich, sweet-tasting pies and puddings. *Yellow squash, zucchini,* and other summer varieties are light and appetizing.

Health Benefits: Squashes are nourishing for the pancreas, spleen, and stomach and give calm, centering energy. They are used in sweet vegetable drink, azuki-squash-kombu, and other medicinal dishes. They are high in beta-carotene (vitamin A).

Recipe for Creamy Squash Soup: Wash and peel 1 large butternut squash. Cut into 1-inch chunks and put in a pan. Add spring water to partially cover. Bring to a boil, reduce heat, and simmer until tender, about 10-20 minutes. Remove and purée in a food mill. Add more water to desired thickness. Return to pan, add 1-2 tsp. of shoyu to taste, and simmer for several minutes. Serve with chopped parsley or scallions.

Cost: Assorted $.75-1.00 lb.; peak autumn-winter

Composition of Butternut Squash, 100 Grams, Edible Portion

Water 86.4 gm.	Calories 45	Protein 1.0 gm.	Fat 0.1 gm.	Carbo. 11.7 gm.	Fiber 1.5 gm.	Calcium 48 mg.	Phos. 33 mg.
Iron 0.7 mg.	Sodium 4 mg.	Potass. 352 mg.	Vit. A 7800 I.U	Thiamin 0.10mg	Ribofla. 0.02 mg.	Niacin 1.2 mg.	Vit. C 21 mg.

TEMPEH

Tempeh, made from fermented soybeans, has a rich, dynamic taste. Originally from Indonesia, it has now encircled the world.

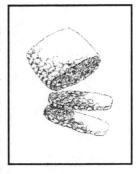

Varieties & Use: Tempeh can be made at home or be purchased ready-made, plain or mixed with brown rice, millet, or other grain. This versatile food can be steamed, pan-fried, boiled, broiled, and deep-fried. Sliced in small quares or rounds, it is enjoyed plain or cooked with grains, vegetables, or seaweed.

Health Benefits: As a fermented soyfood, tempeh is associated with reducing cholesterol, preventing and relieving cancer, and strengthening the kidneys, bladder, and reproductive organs. It is high in protein, calcium, iron, and B vitamins and is a primary plant-quality source of vitamin B_{12}.

Recipe for Tempeh Melt: Cut 8 oz. of tempeh into chunks and cook in a small volume of spring water in a sauce pan for 20-30 minutes. Add sauerkraut to cover, shoyu to taste, and a thick layer of grated mochi (direct from the package). Cook 5-7 minutes or until done.

Cost: $1.25-1.75/8 oz. package; year-round

Composition of Tempeh, 100 Grams, Edible Portion

Water	Calories	Protein	Fat	Carbo.	Fiber	Calcium	Phos.
55.0 gm.	199	19.0 gm.	7.7 gm.	17.0 gm.	--	93 mg.	206 mg.
Iron	Sodium	Potass.	Vit. A	Thiamin	Ribofla.	Niacin	Vit. B_{12}
2.3 mg.	6 mg	367 mg.	686 I.U.	0.13 mg.	0.11 mg.	4.6 mg.	1.0 mcg.

TOFU

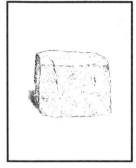

Tofu (also known as *soybean curd*) has a soft texture, mild taste, and versatile shape that combines well with many foods.

Varieties & Use: Home-made tofu is fresh and satisfying. Store-bought tofu comes in several forms: *regular, firm* or hard, *silky* or soft, and *spiced*. Tofu can be steamed, sautéed, boiled, baked, tempuraed, or deep-fried. It is enjoyed plain, used in soups, stews, stir-fries, noodle dishes, sandwiches, and sauces and dressings. Children like scrambled tofu. *Dried tofu*, made from thin dry cakes, gives a unique texture and taste.

Health Benefits: Tofu is an excellent source of protein, calcium, iron, vitamin A, and B vitamins. It is very digestible and contributes to better circulation, respiration, and nervous functioning. A *tofu plaster* is used to bring down inflammation, swellings, and bruises and is more effective than ice.

Recipe for Boiled Tofu: Place 8 oz. of tofu, sliced in pieces 1/2-inch thick, in a pot with 1/4-inch of water and bring to a boil. Reduce heat, simmer for 1-2 min., and serve with a sauce made by mixing spring water, shoyu, and grated fresh ginger. Pour 1 tsp. sauce over each slice and garnish with parsley or scallions.

Cost: Fresh $1.00-1.50/lb.; Dried $6.00/3.5 oz.; year round

Composition of Fresh Tofu, 100 Grams, Edible Portion

Water	Calories	Protein	Fat	Carbo.	Fiber	Calcium	Phos.
84.6 gm.	76	8.1 gm.	4.8 gm.	1.9 gm.	1.2 gm.	105 mg.	97 mg.
Iron	Sodium	Potass.	Vit. A	Thiamin	Ribofla.	Niacin	Vit. C
5.4 mg.	7 mg	121 mg.	85 I.U.	0.08 mg.	0.05 mg.	0.2 mg.	0.1 mg.

TURNIP GREENS

Turnip greens, one of the most nutritious leafy vegetables, are sacred to the American South. They grow in all climates and have a soft, delicate texture and delectable taste.

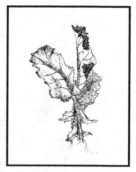

Varieties & Use: Turnip greens are available in the natural foods store or farmers market and are readily grown in the garden. They are enjoyed as a small side dish (cooked by themselves or with turnip roots). They can also be added to soups and salads.

Health Benefits: Turnip greens are loaded with calcium, iron, dietary fiber, and vitamins A and C. They help to strengthen the blood, tonify the liver and gallbladder, and prevent bone loss. Home remedies include *leafy greens juice* and as a substitute for daikon leaves in a *hip bath*. They can also be used as a *cholorophyl plaster* to bring down fever and inflammations and relieve burns and bruises.

Recipe for Turnip Greens with Sesame-Shoyu Sauce: Place 3 cups sliced turnip greens in 1/4-1/2-inch of boiling water. Cover and boil for 2-3 min. Stir occasionally to cook evenly. Roast 2 Tbsp. sesame seeds and grind slightly. Add a little shoyu and water to make a sauce and mix in with greens or serve at table.

Cost: $1.00-2.00/lb.; peak autumn-winter

Composition of Turnip Greens, 100 Grams, Edible Portion

Water 91.1 gm.	Calories 27	Protein 1.5 gm.	Fat 0.3 gm.	Carbo. 5.7 gm.	Fiber 3.2 gm.	Calcium 190 mg.	Phos. 42 mg.
Iron 1.1 mg.	Sodium 40 mg.	Potass. 296 mg.	Vit. A 7600 IU.	Thiamin 0.07 mg.	Ribofla. 0.1 mg.	Niacin 0.6 mg.	Vit. C 60 mg.

UMEBOSHI PLUMS

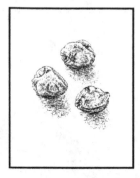

Umeboshi, a salty, pickled plum, has a tangy flavor, combining a sour and salty taste, and has a wide range of culinary and medicinal uses.

Varieties & Use: Related to the apricot, umeboshi plums grow in the warmer, southern and middle regions of Japan and California. *Whole plums* are used as a condiment, a seasoning, and inserted in the center of rice balls. *Ume paste* is a purée made from the pitted plums and is used for convenience to make sauces, dressings, and spreads (delicious on corn on the cob). *Shiso* (or *beefsteak leaves*), the deep red or purple leaves umeboshi are pickled with, make a condiment for grains, soups, or vegetables.

Health Benefits: Umeboshi has a balanced, centering energy that neutralizes extreme foods and conditions. As a fermented food, whole plums aid in digestion, strengthen the blood, and neutralize acidity. Umeboshi are used in *ume-sho-kuzu* drink, and *ume extract*, a concentrate, is used medicinally.

Recipe for Umeboshi Spread: Purée 1-2 plums in a mortar with a little water or corn oil (or use ume paste) and apply lightly to corn on the cob. It's salty, so use moderately.

Cost: $10.00/6 oz.; $20.00/1 lb.; Paste $6.50/6 oz.

Composition of Umeboshi Plums, 100 Grams, Edible Portion

Water 69.8 gm.	Calories 17	Protein 0.3 gm.	Fat 0.8 gm.	Carbo. 3.4 gm.	Fiber 0.3 gm.	Calcium 6.1 mg.	Phos. 26 mg.
Iron 2.0 mg.	Sodium 9400 mg	Potass. --	Vit. A 0	Thiamin 0.06 mg.	Ribofla. 0.09 mg.	Niacin 0.6 mg.	Vit. C 0

WAKAME

Wakame, a sea vegetable gathered off coastal Japan, China, and Korea, turns a beautiful, translucent green when cooked.

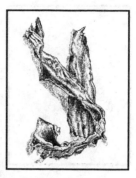

Varieties & Use: Wild and domesticated varieties are available imported from the Far East. *Alaria,* a similar plant, is harvested from the Atlantic off the coasts of the U.S. and the British Isles and Scandinavia. Wakame is popular in miso soup. It is also enjoyed as a small side dish with onions or scallions and goes well with carrots, cauliflower, parsnips, burdock, celery, daikon, and cabbage. It is usually seasoned with shoyu.

Health Benefits: Wakame is high in calcium, iron, vitamin A, B vitamins, and iodine. It helps protect against high blood pressure, prevent tumors, and offset radiation.

Recipe for Wakame with Onions: Wash 1 oz. of dried wakame, soak 3-5 minutes, and slice down the thick center vein lengthwise and then into 1-inch pieces. Place in a pot next to 2 medium-sized onions, peeled and sliced. Add soaking water to almost cover the sea vegetable. Bring to a boil, reduce the heat to low, and simmer for 30 minutes or until tender. Add shoyu, 1-2 tsp., to taste and cook for 10-15 minutes longer.

Cost: $5.00/1.76-2 oz.; year-round

Composition of Wakame, 100 Grams, Edible Portion

Water	Calories	Protein	Fat	Carbo.	Fiber	Calcium	Phos.
13.0 gm.	--	15.0 gm.	3.2 gm.	35.3 gm.	2.7 gm.	960 mg.	400 mg.
Iron	Sodium	Potass.	Vit. A	Thiamin	Ribofla.	Niacin	Vit. C
7.0 mg.	6100 mg	5500 mg	1800 IU	0.30 mg.	1.15 mg.	8.0 mg.	15

WATERCRESS

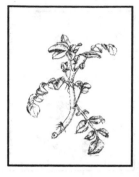

Native to Asia, Europe, and North America, watercress has a bright green color, pungent, slightly bitter taste, and soft texture that makes it a popular leafy green in salads, soups, and other dishes.

Varieties & Use: Watercress comes in *curly* and *straight leaf* varieties. Cooking softens its strong flavor, brights its color, and creates a crisp, refreshing taste. Watercress salads are enjoyed with a creamy tofu or sesame dressing. Steamed watercress seasoned with shoyu is known in Japan as *oshitashi*. Watercress rolls, wrapped with toasted nori, are tasty.

Health Benefits: Watercress is high in calcium, vitamins A and C, and other nutrients. Its fiber aids in digestion. Watercress is especially strengthening to the liver and gallbladder. As an external remedy, it can be used to make a *chlorophyll plaster* or a *potato-leafy greens plaster*.

Recipe for Boiled Watercress: Wash 1 bunch of watercress well. Bring 1/4-inch of spring water to a boil and add half the watercress. Cook for 30-40 seconds, moving it around gently to ensure even cooking. Remove, drain, and repeat with the remaining watercress. Garnish with sesame seeds.

Cost: $1.25-1.50/bunch; year-round

Composition of Watercress, 100 Grams, Edible Portion

Water 95.1 gm.	Calories 11	Protein 2.3 gm.	Fat 0.1 gm.	Carbo. 1.3 gm.	Fiber 1.5 gm.	Calcium 120 mg.	Phos. 60 mg.
Iron 0.2 mg.	Sodium 41 mg.	Potass. 330 mg.	Vit. A 4700 IU.	Thiamin 0.09 mg.	Ribofla. 0.12 mg.	Niacin 0.2 mg.	Vit. C 43 mg.

WHEAT

Wheat is native to Europe, Asia, and the Middle East. Today it is the main grain in North America and China and prized for its flour with which to make bread, noodles, pasta, dumplings, and baked goods.

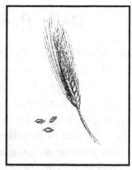

Varieties & Use: *Whole wheat berries* are added to rice and other grains and make a chewy dish. Processed forms of wheat include *cracked wheat, bulgur,* and *couscous.* *Spelt* and *kamut* are heirloom strains of wheat sold under their traditional names. *Hard wheat* contains more gluten than *soft wheat*. *Durum wheat* is used in making pasta and noodles. *Spring* and *winter* varieties indicate time of harvest. *Pastry flour* is used in baking and in tempura batter. (See also *Seitan.*)

Health Benefits: Wheat is high in protein, fiber, calcium, iron, and B vitamins. Whole wheat berries are strengthening to the liver and gallbladder. Wheat flour is used as a stabilizing agent in many home remedies.

Recipe for Brown Rice with Wheat Berries: Wash (and preferably soak 6-8 hours) 1 3/4 cups of brown rice and 1/4 cup whole wheat berries. Pressure cook with a pinch of sea salt for 50 minutes. Garnish with sesame seeds or chopped parsley.

Cost: Wheat Berries $.50-.75/lb.; year-round

Composition of Hard Red Winter Wheat, 100 Grams

Water	Calories	Protein	Fat	Carbo.	Fiber	Calcium	Phos.
13.1 gm.	327	12.6 gm.	1.5 gm.	71.2 gm.	12.2 gm.	29 mg.	288 mg.
Iron	Sodium	Potass.	Vit. A	Thiamin	Ribofla.	Niacin	Vit. E
3.2 mg.	2 mg.	363 mg.	0	0.38 mg	0.12 mg.	5.5 mg.	1.4 mg.

Appendix
Standard Macrobiotic Diet
Daily Foods (in a Temperate Climate)

Whole Cereal Grains
On the average, 50 percent of daily intake by weight should include cooked, organically grown, whole cereal grains, which may be pre-pared in a variety of ways. These include brown rice, millet, oats, corn, rye, wheat, buckwheat, and others. A portion of this amount may consist of noodles or pasta, unyeasted whole grain breads, and other processed grains or grain products. However, whole grain pre-pared in whole form should ideally form the center of every meal.

Soups
About 5 to 10 percent of our daily food (1 to 2 cups or bowls) may in-clude soup made with vegetables, sea vegetables (such as wakame or kombu), grains, or beans. Seasonings include miso, shoyu (natural soy sauce), and sea salt.

Vegetables
About 25 to 30 percent of our daily food consists of vegetables, locally and organically grown whenever possible. Vegetables may be cooked in various styles: steaming, boiling, sautéed with a small amount of sesame oil, and occasionally deep-fried or baked as health permits. A small portion may be eaten occasionally as fresh raw salad and frequently as boiled or pressed salad.

Beans and Sea Vegetables
About 5 to 10 percent of daily diet includes cooked beans and sea veg-etables. Bean products such as tofu, tempeh, and natto may be used daily. Sea vegetables such as nori, wakame, and kombu are recom-mended for daily use.

Seasonings and Condiments
Seasonings are used to enhance flavor and taste and are recommend-ed for use in moderate amounts. Seasonings to be used daily include unrefined white sea salt with a balanced mineral content, traditional-ly made miso that has aged two or more years, and natural shoyu.

They should be cooked with the foods, not added at the table. Cooking oil should be vegetable quality only, especially unrefined sesame oil (light or dark) or unrefined corn oil. Condiments allow for individual variety and taste. They are kept on the table and used, if desired.

Pickles
A small amount of pickles traditionally made from the highest quality ingredients are eaten daily with meals. A variety of pickles are recommended including sauerkraut, miso, shoyu, and umeboshi pickles.

Beverages
Recommended daily beverages include roasted bancha twig tea, roasted brown rice tea, and roasted barley tea. Any traditional tea that does not have an aromatic fragrance or a stimulating effect may be used. For drinking or cooking, good quality water (preferably natural spring or well water) may be used.

Supplemental Foods

Fish and Seafood
Fresh low-fat, white-meat fish such as cod, flounder, or sole once or twice a week in modest volume. Fish may be prepared in a variety of ways, especially steaming, boiling, poaching, or lightly sautéing. Fatty red-meat, blue-skinned, and shellfish are used sparingly.

Fruit
Fruit, including fresh, dried, and cooked fruits, may be taken two to three times a week. Local and organically grown fruits are prefered, such as apples, cherries, pears, peaches, apricots, berries, and melons.

Seeds and Nuts
Nuts and seeds such as pumpkin seeds, sesame seeds, sunflower seeds, peanuts, walnuts, and pecans may be enjoyed as a snack. Other snacks include mochi, sushi, rice cakes, and popcorn.

Natural Desserts
Naturally sweetened desserts such as puddings, natural gelatins, cakes, pies, puddings, and cookies may be taken several times a week as health permits. These should be made with good quality ingredients (no eggs, refined flour, or dairy) and naturally sweetened with amasake, barley malt, or rice syrup or, occasionally, fruit juice.

Recipe Index